COULDN'T HAPPEN TO ME

A LIFE CHANGED BY PARALYSIS AND TRAUMATIC BRAIN INJURY

JILL C. MASON

ISBN: 1-4392-4035-3
ISBN-13: 9781439240359
LCCN: 2009904426

Visit www.booksurge.com to order additional copies.

For Joanne, Larry, and Dan: My mom, dad, and brother who may have lost hope from time to time but never gave up.

And, most of all, for Alan.

ABOUT THE AUTHOR

Jill Mason was 26 in 2004 when she was hit by a drunk driver in Santa Rosa, California, as she was riding her bike in preparation for an upcoming triathlon. Her boyfriend, Alan Liu, was killed outright. With a newly-minted master's degree in communications, Jill worked for an engineering firm and pursued her love of athletics. She played lacrosse for Santa Clara University, from which she graduated in 1999. She was a champion high school runner in Grass Valley, California, where she grew up--and to where she returned after the accident when she was unable to take care of herself. Although she remained in a coma for months, through extraordinary determination, hard work, and loving care, she has managed to begin to live independently in Sacramento.

Jill gives speeches to new cadets in the California Highway Patrol, talks with students all over northern California in the "Every 15 Minutes" program, and in 2008 was selected through a competitive essay contest to be an Olympics torchbearer. She continues to take adaptive physical education classes at Sacramento City College and is a volunteer with physical therapy students at California State University-Sacramento.

Author's Note

I have been working on this book for a number of years. Because of my head injury, my memory and my writing style have changed (improved!) as time has passed. I apologize for my occasional haphazard repetition, but it does illustrate the effects of my head injury. Please keep this in mind when you are reading my story, and please don't get frustrated! All the book comes straight out of my head except parts covering the accident itself, Santa Rosa Memorial Hospital, and early days at Santa Clara Valley Medical Center--of those times I have no memory at all. All of what is written about those horrible days was cobbled together from family, friends, website posts, and a journal my family kept. Most of the quotations were marked by me in Bartlett's Familiar Quotations long before the accident. I would like to thank my friends Sarah and Jen and my family for their editorial help and my aunt Carol for being such an understanding and patient main editor!

JILL C. MASON

Sacramento, California
June 2009

Editor's Note

Exactly five years ago, my sister and I stood over the bed of our badly broken niece, Jill. She looked like nothing more than a wounded bird, her big brown eyes full of fear, startling easily. At the end of a long day in what turned out to be the second worst week of her life--the first being that in which she had been hit by a drunk driver--we shouted at her to look at us. She only looked stunned. Her beautiful hair had been shaved from half her head, her legs were useless, her fist and arm were clenched, and her front tooth was chipped. From that day to today, she has pushed herself, literally, and accomplished a hard-won independence, mobility in her beloved red car, and the writing and publication of this book. She may struggle with a memory that lets her down and legs that no longer carry her around a track, but she has not lost a scintilla of her sparkle or an iota of her fierce determination. She is a hard-working miracle. There is no one in the world I admire more.

Carol L. Mason

Annapolis, Maryland
June 2009

Table of Contents

Part Two: Life Begins

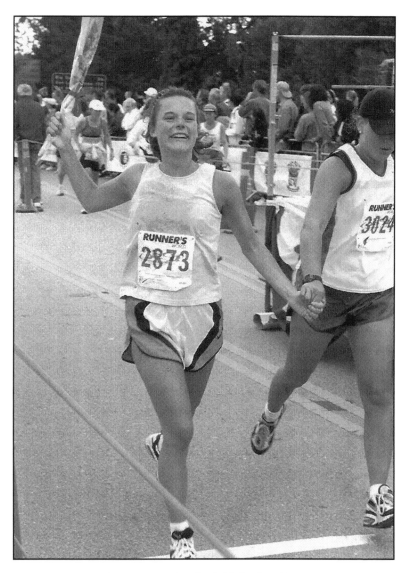

Jill Mason and her friend Liz crossing the finish line in a Big Sur marathon, 1999.

CHAPTER ONE

WHAT HAPPENED

Is it so small a thing
To have enjoyed the sun,
To have lived light in the spring,
To have loved, to have thought, to have done,
To have advanced true friends,
and beat down baffling foes?

Matthew Arnold, Empedocles on Etna, 1852, act II, l 397

Late Easter morning in California in 2004, a sad, drunk old man turned left onto Santa Rosa's Highway 12 from Pythian Road, near where he lived. Weaving, Harvey Hereford swerved onto the shoulder, hit something that shattered his windshield, but he kept on going until he hit something else, and still he kept on going. About three hundred feet down the highway, he finally came to a complete stop, unable to see from inside his aging Nissan what incredible destruction he had left in his wake.

Two bicyclists were on their way home from a quick training session for the upcoming Wildflower Half Ironman Triathlon in California's Lake San Antonio before sitting down with the family for an Easter lunch. The bicyclist in the rear, Alan Liu, was killed instantly. The second cyclist had her spine snapped like a twig in the impact. Motorists stopped and comforted her, crying and shaking, as they waited for the ambulance. Someone else clamped onto Harvey, who still didn't really know what he'd done.

I was the second cyclist, and I don't remember any of this.

Some of what I know now came from the news reports—the local *Press Democrat* and the *San Francisco Chronicle* covered the story; some came from the police reports. Most of what I know about that morning comes from my family and friends telling me what happened. To be on the safe side, no one told me about Alan's death until a long time afterward. In fact, they waited to say anything about his death until I could respond. For a long time I couldn't even remember much of the six months before the accident, which may have spared me some early grief because it was during those six months when I fell in love with Alan.

I come from a huge, very close Italian-Irish family that celebrates holidays and birthdays together often, so I spent Saturday night and Easter morning at my Grammy Carbone's house in San Rafael. My mom and dad were there from Grass Valley, and my brother Dan, who is three years younger, was there from Pleasanton. I woke each of them to say goodbye before driving up to meet Alan in Santa Rosa at his mother Rita's and his stepfather Dane's house. Because we were training for Wildflower, scheduled for early May, we decided to go on a bike ride on Highway 12 before eating Easter brunch. We were both wearing our helmets, as we always did.

We loved to ride—a good thing for triathletes who also need to love running and swimming. We rode a couple of times a week together mid-day from Mountain View on the many good trails just off Foothill Expressway, one of the roads that runs through Silicon Valley. Weekends, we rode up to Stanford University snaking on Skyline through the foothills between Lexington Reservoir and Half Moon Bay. We'd spent a recent weekend in Lake San Antonio with a bunch of other friends who had signed up for the race in May. About ten of us rented a mobile home on the lake; the long weekend was filled with riding and swimming.

Alan's mom, Rita Wells, told me later that I was wearing my biking clothes when I arrived. Sometimes I think, if only I had taken the time to change at their house, maybe Harvey would have made his turn, maybe he would have driven into a quiet ditch somewhere, and Alan and I would have missed our fate. But it is silly to play the "what if" game.

I rode in front of Alan. To this day, I'm not sure why I was leading. My only thought is that I could set the slower pace for us because Alan was a stronger rider. From what the police reports said, we were about

100 feet apart in the bike lane of the road. We were hit from behind at 11:29 a.m. by a car driven by a man whose blood-alcohol level was nearly four times the legal limit. He was driving a Nissan Sentra—the same kind of car in which I learned to drive. Alan was declared dead once they found him off the road, and I was severely hurt.

The only reason Harvey Hereford stopped was because he could not see through his shattered windshield. A few drivers saw the collision and stopped to do what they could. Two women rushed to put blankets over me to try to stop the uncontrollable shaking, and they stayed with me for the time it took the ambulance to arrive. Others who stopped--at least one an off-duty police officer--made sure Harvey, the man who hit us, did not drive away. People told me that Alan was not found until the paramedics arrived.

Traffic on Highway 12 was stopped for a few hours. The paramedics took me to Santa Rosa Memorial Hospital in an ambulance. Rita was listening to the radio and heard the news report about the accident. We were late for brunch, and she knew immediately exactly who the two bicyclists were.

Rita looked for my cell phone and scrolled to see the numbers I had called most recently. Not surprisingly, my brother Dan's number came up first. When Rita phoned, he had just left Grammy's in San Rafael. He got the terrible news that his sister was near death in the hospital in Santa Rosa and immediately turned his car around and drove back to Grammy's house. He frantically knocked on the door and then collapsed on the front porch, too weak to stand. My

80-plus-year-old grandmother took one look at her always competent, can-handle-anything grandson, and told him to get in her car. To this day, I am so glad he went to Grammy's for help rather than trying to drive directly to the hospital in Santa Rosa. She would drive to the hospital. She knew he couldn't.

Dan called our parents, Larry and Joanne Mason. They had started up toward home on Highway 101 from San Rafael before getting the horrible call. They just kept driving north–weeping, screaming, hysterical–praying that their only daughter would still be alive when they got to the Santa Rosa hospital. They tried hard not to think about how she might look or even if they would be able to see her. They drove. They later remembered absolutely nothing about getting to the hospital or what happened first when they did get there.

. . .

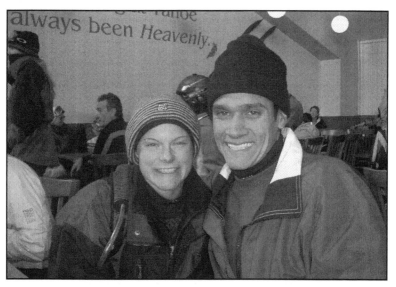

Jill and Alan at Lake Tahoe's Heavenly Ski Resort in 2003.

CHAPTER TWO

BEFORE THE ACCIDENT: ALAN

"Love is the only game not called on account of darkness."
Anonymous

When one of Alan's fellow coaches on the Mountain View Masters swim team heard about the accident, he said the team could have filled the pool with their tears. I had no tears for him then—I couldn't remember that he was my boyfriend, and I didn't even know he died until I read an email four months later about the accident. I remember now.

We meet when I joined the Mountain View Masters swim team in September 2003. I am 26, he is 31, and I suffer uncharacteristic hot flashes at the sight of him, shaking of my voice and hands, and a bad case of junior-high-school shyness. Every Monday, Wednesday, and Friday I drive into the parking lot anxious to see his slim figure poolside in his Euro shoes. Just in case we actually speak, I wear my cutest clothes, even though it's so early, and I brush my hair and teeth with great care.

Before he opens his mouth, I love the way he moves, the way he demonstrates the drills. The rhythm drives me mad-out-of-mind. His energy is a magnet and makes me laugh louder, become giddier (and it's only 7:07 a.m.!), as I walk through the pool gates. As my family will quickly point out, I'm not much of a morning person, but this feeling made all of that go away. I like his white broad smile. His hands. His voice. His incredible brown eyes.

Besides coaching the team, Alan is a mechanical engineer devoted to his work and his profession—not an "enginerd," as he sometimes describes several of his MIT classmates and coworkers. Alan is motivated, witty, athletic, energetic, and loves his cat.

I have the crush of all crushes. My mom observes that this is the first time in a long time I've admitted being attracted to someone. I think she's counseling some restraint, but I know that I'm more than willing to make a fool out of myself for this guy if he's available.

I admire him from afar until I think about actually

entering a swim meet, and I email him for my estimated times. He writes back!!! And he's a great writer. Amazing. A man who can express himself in writing is so very sexy. Another excuse to interact with this fellow: he finds out about my Lake of the Pines Triathlon race results and posts them on the swim team website. I proudly show him my competition-scraped knees in the pool afterwards.

He makes me utterly absentminded, and I leave ALL my shower gear and bathing suit and goggles in the shower one Friday morning. Incredible luck: He's at the pool on a Saturday afternoon when I return to pick up my gear from the lost-and-found! Even luckier, I'm wearing a little jean skirt and my cute Spanish sandals rather than my typical thesis-writing grubbies! Oh, but how idiotic and mindless I feel retrieving absolutely EVERYTHING that's supposed to be in my swim bag, especially with him breathing over my shoulder as we look under the desk together.

In September, after the San Francisco T-Mobile bike race, I'm eating pizza in a restaurant with my friend Erin, my brother Daniel, and his friend. Here comes Alan into the restaurant. Erin recognizes him, and Daniel whispers across the table: Is this THE swim coach you told us about? I nod and curse, with my mouth full, feeling the heat crawl up my neck. Chew, chew, I tell myself, so you can introduce him to your BROTHER and HIS friend Geoff. I am not on a date, I'm desperate to say. Relax, for crying out loud, he's probably married. BUT, just in case he's not, make it perfectly clear you are by no means on a double date. Alan has a permanent pen-number still visible on his calf from a triathlon in Pacific Grove the day before. I ask him about the triathlon. He seems taken aback at first, surprised I would know about the event, and then says he did well in his age group. I only know you were racing, I think, because of my laser-like focus on your legs. I'm not stalking you, really!

I'm sure he's married, or at least wildly unavailable, and my crush turns to agony. But he speaks to me, and he even seeks me out sometimes. I am speechless and hopeless. A few weeks prior to the first date: Drill, kick, swim, breathe, swim, breathe, rest, kick, hop out of pool. Walk towards locker room . . . oh, he's walking toward me. Oh my, he's turning to cross my path. Oh god! He's walking this way. What do I say? Aaaah! He speaks. I am stunned, like a deer in the headlights but determined to be myself. After the encounter, I hope I didn't say anything weird because I can't remember anything either of us said. In my mind, I silently celebrate in the shower!

Finally, he asks me if I am going to celebrate my second-place finish at the Lake of the Pines Triathlon. Totally clueless, I say I am going out to dinner with friends on two different nights that week. He drops the bomb (as I almost drop my goggles and fall over) asking, "Can I take you out sometime?" Gulp. Uh, excuse me? I think I hear him right, but I blurt out that I think he's married. He laughs and says, no, that he's not. I'm elated, shaking even, in the shower, can't stop smiling like a dope. I call my mom, my friends Kina and Becky, and my brother Daniel on the way to work (during the seven-minute commute), and I don't get a thing done at work that day.

And that's how everything started: The runner and swimmer and biker Jill Christine Mason met the swimmer and runner and biker Alan Barry Liu. I grew up in a little town called Grass Valley, but was born in Lincoln, Nebraska, and went to Santa Clara University and San Jose State for graduate school. He grew up in the Oakland hills, went to Massachusetts Institute of Technology and then Stanford for graduate school. I was working in marketing communications for an engineering company; he was an engineer. We both loved each other, music, athletics, and our cats—his was Emma, mine was Charlie. We both had, and I still have, lots of energy to share.

I was still pitifully nervous when we met at a restaurant in downtown Mountain View for our first date, but then I saw he was, too, so I settled down and focused on being myself. We had a great time! I wrote my brother Dan that I thought he was a keeper, and I told him everything I'd found out during our four-hour date: he had been swimming competitively all his life, played golf, traveled in Italy one summer using books about Italian wineries as a guide; was on the varsity water polo and swimming teams at MIT and earned his master's in mechanical engineering from Stanford. He had been at Applied Materials in Silicon Valley for eight years. Alan was a huge sports fan of the Raiders, unfortunately. In spite of that, he was, in short, perfect. We made our next date—running at Rancho San Antonio—that night.

Alan also loved his cars and his wine, both conveniently housed in his carport. He had a silver BMW 2002 with the license plate "ABL 2002" and a green Bronco. Once we went to Calistoga with his friends Paul and Dotty. We both brought our road bikes and running clothes and rode our bikes from winery to winery. He knew one of the wine makers at Olabisi Winery, and we had a private tasting in the cellar with the owner. (I shared the last bottle of Olabisi Wine with my girlfriends just a few months ago, more than five years later.)

We often went to dinner together at the great restaurants in Mountain View, especially Yakko, a place that serves sushi. The restaurant has tables with a bench on each side connected to the wall. The person who sits against the wall, facing the kitchen, needs to climb into the seat. On one of our first dates there, Alan gave me a Foxtrot comic he cut out of the paper, slightly edited as follows: "I'm thinking I'd like to run a marathon with Jill. You should call Alex Bixby's husband then. He runs marathons with Jill? He sells life insurance." This kind of comedy was so Alan. He especially liked giving funny award to his swimmers, awards like: *Best Runner Pretending to be a Swimmer, Most Punctual Award, Best Suit, etc.*

Alan had this way of tipping his head back and laughing whole-heartedly. I loved his laugh; it was infectious. I have a digital video my parents, Alan, and I took of Dan when he was competing in a bike race at Mather Field in Sacramento in February 2004. I caught the sound of Alan's laugh on my digital video, and I love to hear it. Sometimes I can still see him walking along the pool deck, carrying his thermos as the team members swam, sipping his coffee that he kept on the ladder of the high diving board, laughing from the bottom up, demonstrating the swimming drills, and loving life.

I often think that he is watching me and making sure my life is as good as possible. I always picture what it would be like with him there. When I'm with my family and friends, I keep thinking, even now, many years later, 'Alan would have loved this!' Watching my cousins play in the pool always makes me think of how much Alan would love to be doing the same. I wish we'd had more time, but we didn't.

· · ·

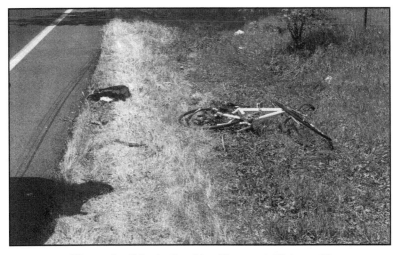

Jill's wrecked bike by the side of Sonoma's Highway 12.

CHAPTER THREE

VIGIL AT THE SANTA ROSA MEMORIAL HOSPITAL (APRIL 11-MAY 11, 2004)

"Enjoy the little things, for one day you may discover they were the big things."

Anonymous

Of course I remember absolutely nothing of Santa Rosa Memorial hospital, but within three days of the accident, friends from work launched my website, www.jillmason.com, so any updates or news could be posted. The website chronicled those terrible days. Some of what follows comes from that record, but more comes from my parents and their own notes.

The second night after I was hit, the Santa Rosa Bike Coalition held a candlelight vigil in the front of the hospital, a show of concern from complete strangers that my family found touching and helpful. They just lit candles and watched them burn. No one said a word, although they were available to talk if my parents approached them. Betsy and Rusty Dillon turned up to tell my parents about their son's horrific brain injury cause by a driver-biker accident like mine and his continued slow recovery. I think they offered one painfully thin shred of hope.

Far more powerful, though, was the huge group that showed up at the hospital, what my friends described as the "Jill Mason fan club that was beyond primo." My large family naturally fills out a lot of the numbers, but I'm lucky to have so many friends. My parents let them see me "sleeping" and on a respirator, and my colleague Danh wrote on the website of how hard it was to see me lying still; "In all the time that we have known her, she has never been still for more than 0.8 of a second."

The outlook was desperate in those first few hours—I was unresponsive when I arrived at the hospital. The trauma doctor and the neurosurgeon took my parents and brother into a small conference room when they arrived. He proceeded to brief them on the long list of critical injuries that I had sustained. Each description was delivered with the big caveat:

"If she survives." The first, and most critical problem was widespread severe traumatic brain injury. I was suffering many small infarcts or strokes in my brain, and there were indications of major damage to the brain stem and cerebellum. My mother wrote in a small notebook someone thoughtfully provided that the suggestion would probably be made to "pull the plug." "If survives," she continued scribbling, "functional level is comatose—could get pneumonia." After saying this, the doctor explained that my spine had been fractured in at least three locations and had been completely dislocated at the T-12 level. This dislocation led them to believe, with high confidence, that my spinal cord was not just dislocated but completely severed at that level. In addition to these two highly critical injuries, I had a long list of other issues: a puncture wound to the liver, rib fractures including lung bruising, a severe fracture to the left wrist, fractures to heel and foot bones, and many lacerations, abrasions, and contusions. The mind-numbing length of the list seemed unimportant in the face of the most basic fact that my injuries would likely be fatal.

The small notebook swelled with medical updates, questions, and to-do lists. Optimistically, they created a separate section right away: Milestones. Even on that first disastrous day, they noted my pulse and blood pressure were lowering and that I blinked my left eye. Heavily sedated, my father added, maybe hoping this explained it all. They found it impossible to believe I would always be paralyzed and had no comprehension of brain injury. All they wanted was for me to live. The future stretched from hour to hour at that point.

My parents and brother spent the first night in the hospital taking turns at my bedside. With no hopeful signs from the doctors looking over me, they were left to spend their time staring at my battered and sedated body, hoping that I'd wake up and be my same old self at any moment. The more realistic fears were that I could never wake up from the coma into which I had dropped. The doctors finally made them leave at 5 a.m. They tried to sleep in the waiting room for an hour and returned at 6 a.m.

Tubes and machines were everywhere, beeping, blinking and spewing numbers. In addition to the typical vitals on the monitor (heart rate, blood pressure, etc.), I had a hole drilled into my skull which allowed my intracranial pressure to be continuously monitored. My family would spend hours agonizing over every small change in any of these parameters: is that too high? too low? does this number mean she's feeling pain? It was possible for them to torture themselves for hours just staring at the silly monitors.

My face, they said, was swollen beyond recognition and my hair and face matted with dried blood, probably from a huge cut and several smaller ones still visible. Road rash on my right arm was bright and angry. Curiously, the flowers that had been painted on my toenails during my last pedicure were nearly intact; only one was scraped when my bike shoes flew off on impact. My legs, finely tuned for the upcoming triathlon, still looked strong.

On the third day, Tuesday morning, though, the neurosurgeon delivered a sliver of hope. He informed everyone that some of my major brain swelling had gone down and that the critical portions the trauma doctor thought were cut off due to strokes were possibly getting blood flow after all. He detected some sign of activity in my brain as well as indications that the damage initially thought to be fatal was perhaps not to that level. He was concerned about strokes in the cerebellum and trauma to the brain stem, but he asked for a delay of two or three days before discussing his prognosis of future function. My family interpreted this as a positive assessment, At this point the neurosurgeon's warning that I had a high probability of ending up in a "persistent vegetative state" was not something that my family had the emotional capacity to ponder.

The doctor explained that my body had been under severe stress, that high blood pressure, raising arms and shrugging shoulders—unmeaningful movement—were normal reactions. He tossed my parents and brother a small bone, however: blinking my left eye might actually mean something. Wednesday, day four, was much the same as day three, except that I opened both eyes. Trouble was, my pupils had shifted to the side, a sure indication of brain damage. My dad thought I reacted to my mother's voice, though.

The fourth day, the website reported that I was continuing to get better, that I opened both eyes, that my family thought me more responsive. We've always been an optimistic, fiercely determined family, and later I could read that optimism in the website postings. My back was broken, my brain was damaged, my lungs were bruised, I was infected, but the good news, whatever smidgen available, was reported daily.

On April 15, day five, the good-news flash was a confirmation that the doctors believed I was truly responding voluntarily to my family's voices and moving my arms and eyes. Later we weren't so sure, but the belief must have helped my family at the time. On day five, the doctor described meaningful movement I managed: I wiggled my left pointer finger when asked, and blinked my eyes (one for no, two for yes) when asked. My dad wrote that I greeted them in the morning with both eyes open for 15-20 seconds, and that my eyes were more in line, especially the left. They were delighted to see me turn the corners of my mouth down in a frown and to squeeze Daniel's hand. My parents were grasping at anything. It wasn't for another week that I started to squeeze my parents' and brother's hands more consistently. Hope was my family's best friend.

I had tracheotomy surgery to insert a breathing tube on day five. I could still breathe over the tube (over-breathe), but it was more comfortable inserted in my neck instead of my nose. I couldn't talk because the trach blocked all air traveling past my vocal chords, but my brother wrote on the website that I also probably didn't have the mental capacity to put together sentences in any case. Although we didn't know it at the time, the medical assumption was that the trach would likely be permanent.

I also needed a feeding tube inserted directly into my stomach. This replaced the tube through my nose. Two temporary tubes replaced with two permanent ones.

On the sixth day, I was making more eye contact (or what my family perceived as eye contact when they stuck their faces within a foot of mine, and I opened my eyes) and tracking moving targets—like people. I was doing more breathing on my own, and I opened my mouth when asked in the evening. When asked to squeeze a hand, I could use both hands.

A week after the accident, I was taken off the ventilator. Optimistically, my brother thought I was trying to speak, which I couldn't do in any case because of the tracheotomy tube still in my throat. He reported that I was showing some emotion, mostly by scowling at the nurses when they brushed my teeth. The most touching sign that I was alive was that reportedly I smiled twice, once for my grandmother and once for my college friend Heidi. My brother even planned to go back to work the next day to try to clear his thoughts, although my parents did not give up the constant vigil for many, many weeks.

For about a week, I was on a special bed that rotated me until the surgeons could do the back surgery on April 21. My mom said I hated the bed because of the jostling, but it was supposed to improve my circulation. In response to the position changes, I would flex the muscles in my upper body as if bracing for the movement. About this time, my cousin Jessica told me that she and Dan were trying to get me to spit on him, a complicated command. Unthinkable, but they begged. They were desperate–I spat.

Temperature regulation was a big problem—I sweated profusely. The nurses explained that temperature regulation emanates from the lower brain, which had been damaged, and the sweating was called a neurostorm.

Ten days after the accident, April 21, I finally had the surgery to stabilize my spine. My white cell count had been high because of infection, most likely in my lungs, the doctors said, but the count was down early on Wednesday, and they moved ahead. They initially told my family that it would likely take few surgeries to realign my back and fuse the vertebrae.

My spine needed fusing from T4 to L4, and the doctors, Alan Hunstock and Eldan Eichbalm, were attempting to reduce T12 and L1 dislocation with screws and clamps to fuse the spine to nearby bone. They were using a brand new imaging machine to do the surgery that allowed them to see exactly where they were putting their tools in my back. The doctors worked on my severed spinal cord for nearly twelve hours, and the younger, stronger Dr. Eichbalm apparently had to use brute strength to align it. Miraculously, the doctors were able to complete all of the repairs in one surgery. (Does it sound like I'm talking about a car??)

The doctors were extremely happy with their accomplishment—a feat that could have easily resulted in the nicking of the aorta and my bleeding to death immediately. Post-surgery, they excitedly showed my brother Dan, the mechanical engineer, the before-and-after x-rays. Despite their apparent technical success, the surgeons were not optimistic about my recovery. My nerves were damaged badly, and they put my spinal cord back in as best they could. The doctors took my parents and brother into a small room and told them that, despite their beautiful work, things didn't look promising. I would not use my legs again, they said.

For several days, I was generally unresponsive. Even though they had been warned that I was getting the rest I needed after the trauma of the surgery, my brother wrote that they "really long to see [my] eyes." My cell counts were up and down, as was my fever, but my consciousness far less advanced than before the surgery. Daniel even admitted to my having a difficult day on the 24th.

As my unresponsive days wore on, friends held a mass for me at Mission Santa Clara on Sunday, April 25, two weeks after the accident, and a service of prayer and encouragement at Peace Lutheran Church in Grass Valley. My parents and some of my mother's family were able to go to Mission Santa Clara; my father's sister and more of my mom's family attended the Grass Valley service. Alan's memorial service was later held at Stanford, and my parents and some of mom's family were able to attend.

The day after Alan's funeral, the decision was made to send me to Santa Clara Medical Center—which was known for its impressive rehabilitation facilities—when I was stable enough to go. My family was anxious to get me started in specialized treatment, but I was still fighting fevers, oxygen problems, and infections.

My right arm and hand were absolutely rigid; spastic rigidity is related to brain damage. Dan reported that I opened my hand for my mom, a major breakthrough, and actually extended my arm by April 29, eighteen days after the accident.

The weekend Alan and I were supposed to be racing the Wildflower Triathlon, I was still in Santa Rosa Memorial Hospital. Daniel described my three states: sleeping, a real, restful sleep unlike earlier ones; awareness, with eye contact, following motion, and even a few big smiles; and uncomfortable. Typical engineer, he estimated the "uncomfortable" state at around 40-50% of the day. He couldn't tell whether I felt the pain of my injuries, nausea from the medications, or confusion about what was happening. I kept my eyes closed and scowled.

Occasionally I was wheeled outside in a special big chair similar to a bed. The weather was always beautiful, but there was too much stimulation for me. I was overwhelmed by the feel of the sun and the wind. My eyes would glaze over (even more than they already were), and I would sometimes appear to be in more pain. This was true for months to come.

Here was my diagnosis: Basically, paralyzed at the T-12 level with an unknown degree of brain damage. My mom wrote out the details later:

Traumatic Brain Injury with shearing (intracranial pressure 13-15)

T12 Spinal Cord Injury (complete)

Vertebral artery injury

Puncture wound to liver (Grade 1)

Rib fractures and lung bruising

Fracture to left wrist

Fracture to heel and foot bones

Lacerations, abrasions and contusions

For the first few weeks, my family's ability to determine a "bad day" vs. "good day" and "responsive" vs. "unresponsive" was an extremely imprecise ritual. They were constantly struggling to differentiate between meaningful signs of cognitive activity and comatose restlessness. During the time I was in a coma, aside from when heavily sedated, I didn't lie still very long. Instead, I would flex my arms, clench my fists, and make horribly contorted facial expressions. Doctors were constantly telling us that these were typical among comatose patients, but my family and friends insisted on reading more into them. They would spend every day–emotionally drained and sleep deprived–clutching for some indication that the old Jill was in there. After a few initial indications that I could hear them and respond with facial expressions, there was nothing for weeks.

■ ■ ■

CHAPTER FOUR

BEFORE THE ACCIDENT: JILL WORKING

"A pessimist sees the difficulty in every opportunity; an optimist sees the opportunity in every difficulty."
Winston Churchill

Before the accident, I worked as a marketing communications specialist for Lowney Associates, a small environmental engineering firm in Mountain View purchased by TRC during my last year with them. We had a team of geotechnical and environmental engineers who were often brought in to consult on major property transfers and on significant site hazards. I encouraged the engineers to write articles on environmental hazards and geotechnical issues, and I edited their work. Sometimes the topics were of great interest to the general public, and I pitched the stories via press releases to local newspapers; sometimes the story was covered locally. I also was in charge of the website and our communications with clients and new customers. Lowney sent me to graduate school in communications at San Jose State University, and I earned my master's degree the December before being hit. I loved my job.

One of my most pleasant duties was buying the wine we gave our clients each Christmas. Some of the project managers would come with me to Beltramo's in Menlo Park to sample different wines that Gary, a Beltramo's wine connoisseur, selected. We usually picked a syrah or a cabernet sauvignon. Wine no longer tastes good to me, and I miss a good glass of merlot.

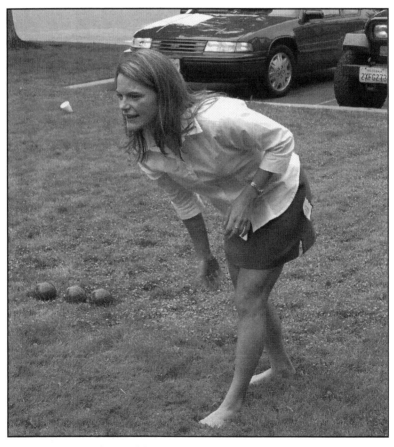

Jill exercising her bocce-ball skills at work.

I had a lot of freedom in my job, and, as long as I accomplished my goals, I could set the pace for my day. Trust was central and worked well for me because I am internally driven. Because I swam Mondays, Wednesdays, and Fridays, I didn't get to work until nine or so. The day was spent editing articles and writing press releases, contacting project managers, working with the print house, AlphaGraphics, and communicating with the Web designer at Tazuma Design.

It was easy marketing such a great firm: they really valued clients' needs as the core of each project. Each project manager took this philosophy to heart, even as he tried to meet the state's or city's requirements while helping a client complete a job. We worked hard to show our clients how important they were to our success; we'd take them to basketball and baseball games, mention their names in press releases, and highlight their important projects in our publications. Clients kept coming back and seemed to respect the work we did. Good thing! I couldn't market a company's product if I didn't believe in it. I am a terrible liar!

We had work parties every quarter to have fun together, meet the new employees, and compare our financial and market status to that of the previous year. We ate, drank, and played bocce ball on the front lawn. The bonus checks were handed out at these parties, with the bonuses based on the firm's profits and employee rank. My points were based on press mentions and anything else I did that could benefit the bottom line.

Some of my closest friends were from Lowney. Just after the accident, Danh, Erin, and Rebecca (who was my predecessor) offered to start jillmason.com so my family could let people know how I was doing. They built the site and posted the first few communiqués, and then my brother took over the updates. It was a blessing for my family not to have to answer telephone calls or individual emails, much as they loved the support of such a vast network of friends and family.

My colleague Danh, also an engineer, often ran with me. He is more of a rider than a runner, and I was more of a runner than a rider, so we were a great team. I never dared ride with him, though, because he was too good for me. Danh had given me his old white road bike, the one I was riding at the time Alan and I were hit. He, his wife, and other Lowney friends and I skied together twice before the accident. We often had lunch together if he was not with a client or at a job site, usually about once a week. I really miss that, but he has assigned me a weekly task: I must call him every Tuesday to catch up. He knows how important repetition is for me now with my head injury.

Another close work friend, Erin, ran with me several times a week at Shoreline Park or Rancho San Antonio so we could stay in shape for triathlon season. She also is a really good rider, and we often met before dawn in Cupertino, riding as the sun rose. Sometimes she met me at my place, and I would scramble out of bed worrying about being late again. She got me started swimming because that is her best event.

Another Lowney friend, Gretchen, joined Danh, Erin and me at least once a month at each other's houses. Danh brought chopsticks for the hostess, whether or not we were eating Chinese. All three brought these chopsticks and my favorite dinner from Bucca di Beppo's to the Santa Clara Valley Medical Center once I was eating again. We remembered a funny dinner at my house just after we found out Danh's wife Mariska was pregnant with their first child, Tyler. As a surprise, Erin and I hid a baby pacifier in the dessert parfait. Thinking he had just bitten down into a terrible cooking mistake, Danh graciously said nothing until we egged him on to dig the pacifier out of the parfait.

Lowney friends and running and swimming and biking and Alan were all thoroughly intertwined. Alan, Erin, and I rode together about twice a week in the middle of the workday, taking the trails just off Foothill Expressway in the Silicon Valley. Sometimes we rode up to Stanford University, snaking through the foothills between Lexington Reservoir and Half Moon Bay on Skyline. Alan drove from his job at Applied Materials in Santa Clara, changed his clothes at home in Mountain View, and biked a half mile to Lowney to meet Erin and me on weekdays. Weekends, we all met in downtown Los Altos to go on longer rides with some other biking friends, including John Nurre, a close friend of ours from the swim team. He wrote me something so poignant that after Alan and I were hit, he kept a photo of Alan taped underneath his bike seat for a year. I love that.

When it looked as if I'd live, my parents let Danh, Erin, and Gretchen see me in the hospital in Santa Rosa. They were the ones who described the situation in the first web posting on April 14: "When we were allowed to see her, she was sleeping and on a respirator. We let her know how much we miss her and that we were thinking of her. It was very difficult to see her in that condition. . . Now to see her lying still like that was very hard."

Danh's old road bike that he gave me was a white Kline. Alan gave me the bike seat, embroidered with a beautiful butterfly on the big part of the seat. We used clipless pedals, special shoes that snap into your pedals and attach you to your bike. The attachment permits more power as the rider's feet come full circle without losing any momentum because the rider's feet push and pull alternately as they spin the pedals. My first time using clipless pedals was not a success. At an intersection in Palo Alto, I couldn't get my foot unclipped quickly enough when I had to stop, and I fell right over onto the sidewalk. I wasn't hurt, but my ego had a bruise.

I loved cycling. Feeling the wind in your face, the power of muscles, the sweat on your brow, it all made me happy. Running was my event, but riding, like swimming, gave my legs a rest from the impact of running. I usually rode for nearly two hours on the weekdays and for three hours on the weekends. Often pedaling 25 to 40 miles in one ride, we covered the foothills of Silicon Valley or rode over the top of Skyline to the Pacific Ocean side to see some of the most glorious views of green pastures, forests, and grassy hills. My brother Dan, Alan, and I took some great rides in Marin County, by Dan's old house in Pleasanton, and outside Livermore.

Erin and Danh and another friend from Lowney, Barry, went ahead and raced the Wildflower Triathlon held in early May for which Alan and I had been practicing. Lots of competitors wore ribbons in memory of Alan and in support of me. Barry wrote an email the day after saying, "yesterday was all about our friend, Jill. . . it was the hardest race I've ever competed in. . . it had to be tough, just like Jill."

My brother Dan didn't compete in Wildflower, though. He is a huge rider. For a time after we were hit, Dan could not get back on his bike. A couple of months after the accident, Dan finally began riding with Danh and Erin. I thank them for taking him under their wings while I was in the hospital. Dan has stayed with riding, thank goodness, and he is only two classes from being a professional cyclist. When he got his new titanium bicycle in 2005, I could even pick it up. I think it weighed 16 pounds.

．　■　■

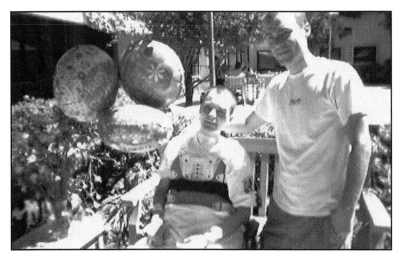

Jill and her brother Dan celebrating her first birthday post-accident, 2004.

CHAPTER FIVE

DESCENDING

"The will to win means nothing without the will to prepare."

Anonymous

My parents were anxious to move me to Santa Clara Valley Medical Center, reputed to be the best place for me to get started on rehabilitation for both my traumatic brain injury (TBI) and spinal cord injury (SCI). Santa Clara would focus first on treating the TBI and provide occupational, physical and speech therapy for at least three months.

The first day planned for the move was May 6 (Day 26),

but a CT scan on May 5 showed that my ventricles continued to enlarge, increasing the pressure on my brain. The move to Santa Clara was immediately delayed. My father noted that I was less alert and sleeping more, and my mom thought my face seemed swollen and my eyes bulging. I was moving my head and my left arm. The doctors had a number of options: wait and see; perform a ventricalostomy, surgically inserting a tube to drain the fluid temporarily; or insert a permanent drainage shunt.

The doctor thought I could manage with the permanent shunt. On May 7, the ventricular-peritoneal shunt was inserted in a bedside surgery, and doctors told my family to expect a change within the week. With relief, my family saw good facial expressions and an improved responsiveness, at least a little, by the next day. Two days after the surgery, I was showing less of a blank stare, but my fever spiked to 105. That night, my father claimed I smiled when he teased me. The next day he put a ball in my gnarled fist and noted in his journal that I dropped the ball. (He seemed to think this was a "milestone," although it doesn't sound promising to me.) He was to keep pushing me—he is a physical education teacher who specializes in working with children with physical challenges—every day, coma or no coma, throughout my long rehabilitation.

I was transferred to the Head Trauma Unit of Santa Clara Valley Medical Center May 11, a month after the accident. For a week, hopes were high that I was progressing steadily and could take advantage of the enormous team assembled for assessment and therapy: speech, occupational, and physical therapists, and a couple of doctors. For the first time, I mouthed the words, "thank you," for which my parents were grateful. Remembered manners and words were a good sign.

Immediately I was given a shot to ease tone in my right arm, and I could extend beyond 90 degrees. The occupational therapists were allowed to prop me in a wheelchair for up to 40 minutes, and I was able to move my neck a little more. The grimaces on my face made it obvious my left side was painful, although I have no recollection of any pain, and I was sweating with any exertion. The nurses were having to suction the mucus from my throat less often, and there was even discussion of using an intermittent (four-to-six hours) catheter for my urine.

Visitors were coming, and I was fairly alert. Sometimes I rolled my eyes in disgust, and my family even thought I was watching television. I shook my head for "no," opened my mouth on command, and continued to open my hand on request. My eyes were tracking far better than they had been.

Two of my mother's sisters are nurses, and they sometimes took the notes in my parents' journal. They were better about tracking all the other problems thriving in the shadow of my brain and spinal injuries. Things like my lacerated liver, yeast in my urine and scalp, and a bladder infections to name a few. Neurosweats (sweating profusely for no apparent reason) were noticeable at this point as well.

One sliver of good news was that my breathing was still pretty good!

The honeymoon ended on Sunday, May 16, five days after my arrival. My left arm tightened, my pulse went up to 150-160 all day, and my fever spiked around noon to 102 degrees. On Monday, the doctors confirmed that my cerebral spinal fluid was infected with "a few organisms," causing my white blood cell count to go up to 28. Nearly finished with an earlier round of antibiotics, I started over again.

I was transferred to the neurological intensive care unit. Very late Wednesday, actually Thursday morning, they took out the shunt, which apparently had never worked properly and was collecting bacteria too tough for antibiotics. A new external shunt was inserted, and a more permanent one would go in a different spot in my skull after a couple of weeks. The pressure on my brain kept going up, and it must have been around this time that I began showing signs of decreased alertness with uneven pupil dilation. The neurosurgeon told my parents that it was unlikely I would ever improve. (Hmm. Maybe he should read this book.) The doctor called my state "coma vigilant."

These were some of the darkest times for my family and friends. After seeing a few token signs of my return to consciousness, I was now just barely clinging to life. Each day the bad news continued to pile up—my vitals were all over the place, and I was deeply unconscious. My room was beautiful and large, overlooking pleasant lawns, but I simply continued to grimace and twitch unnaturally. My mom says she came closest to losing hope during this time. The rehabilitation doctor, Thao Duong, was my strongest advocate–my parents called her an angel of support. We can never thank her enough for her belief in me.

My mom and dad alternated weeks with me, one working back home in Grass Valley and one staying near the medical center. They stayed in my apartment nearby—even continuing to pay the rent because it was less expensive than a hotel. Their schools were very understanding about taking time off, but they still needed to work. My dad pondered asking about early retirement.

My mother's sister, Carr, a nurse, was the official family contact. HIPAA (National Standards to Protect the Privacy of Personal Health Information) laws required a single point of contact. When my parents called from home in Grass Valley to see what kind of a night I had, the nurses were not permitted to say anything, not even whether my temperature was normal. Only Carr could ask. During this particularly dark time at the end of May, my father got frustrated with the requirement and asked to meet with the social worker. He wanted to see the policy that demanded a single point of contact. The social worker didn't produce the policy, and he, usually supremely controlled, started screaming at her because every other word spoken by her was HIPAA. She clearly had no concern for us. The head nurse later agreed to be the contact for either of my parents or my aunt, defusing the whole situation but no doubt putting herself at risk for "breaking the rules."

Another aunt told me that she and her sister (yet another auntie) would stand over my bed and shout, "Look at me! Look at her!" I would startle and turn my head. Sometimes I would even smile, making the whole day worthwhile, she said. Things were so bad at that point, though, many of the therapists weren't coming to work with me. If I were to get help, I would need to show more responses.

My awake coma was very unlike anything you see on TV or in the movies. I did not remember a thing until my birthday—July 9, 2004. I have spotty memories from early on in Santa Clara where I remember brief snippets. But my "waking up" was very gradual. It annoys me when people ask me what it was like to "wake up," because I didn't wake up with any drama. Little things simply got better every day. My family and friends charted every different kind of blink, every different kind of startle, hoping for signs of improvement and increased conscious wakefulness. I did not just wake up, look around, and wonder what the hell had happened. I just inched along, which doesn't make for a very good television script.

My eyes, when they were open, were very glassy, as if someone pulled a sheet across my face. Family and friends say that you could look into my face, and know immediately nobody was home. Even now, when I see photos of me with my cousins, friends, and brother, I can tell how scary it must have been to look at me, with my shaved head, that fragile skull, and that terrible blank stare. Really, I don't have much more to write about because it is all a blank to me. This seems to be a good way to express my memory of my coma: nothing.

Others did have memories of those days, though. Most didn't understand at that time that there were different levels of coma and that someone could still have eyes open yet be considered in a coma. That's why Becky said she didn't remember me being in a coma; she thought I was just sleeping or tired and unresponsive. When she and other friends visited, they would all just sit around and talk to me, telling me stories. Sometimes they gave me pedicures. One time, her co-worker Tisha and she came and they acted out plays for me. They always managed to entertain themselves, and they hoped they entertained me, too. Harder for Becky was looking at the other patients in the head trauma unit. How sad, she thought, as she watched others talking to unresponsive people with no life in their eyes. But they were all positive I was there, sure that I was listening to everything they had to say but just wasn't ready to respond. Somehow no matter how bad it was, they were all sure that I was there. They had to think that to keep up hope. It took many weeks, but they finally got some responses from me to funny stories about school. I was using my eyebrows and eyes to show how involved I was in the stories (mostly embarrassing), and I made lots of faces. That night they asked me if I wanted the light out when they left, and I clearly communicated to them to leave it on. It was the first time she felt hopeful for a good reason.

When my friend from the swim team, Laura, visited me

in the hospital, I was sleeping. She saw how much smaller my legs were and how much smaller I was. I was lying on my side and my head was shaved. Her last memory of me was at the pool and at Lake San Antonio weekend with Alan and other swim team members when we rode bikes and swam. To see me in that state was devastating. She spoke to me, without response, and touched my hand and left feeling very sad and angry. It was really hard for her to see me that way. She wondered, 'How could life change like that for someone like Jill?' Laura was (and still can be) very angry about the situation and the man that put me in this place. She just kept waiting for the day when they had to tell me about Alan and the days when I started to remember him. She was glad I had so much support AND the right kind of support to get me through all of this. She said a feeling came across her that I share: that Alan was with me helping me fight.

My friend Laura from work remembered the constant fear that I wouldn't come out of my coma. One day there would be slight good news, and then the next significant setbacks on the medical front. Daniel was pretty frank with my status on the website. She talked to her family (which includes a number of doctors) about how I was doing, and not all of it was promising. The miracle was I survived the coma state, came out of it, and eventually recovered most of my memories.

No one mentioned Alan for a long time. My family could see that I couldn't even take in what had happened to me, much less to him. My brother wrote that "It occasionally appears that, during brief moments of alertness, she becomes aware that something has gone terribly wrong–but that is probably the extent of her understanding."

∎ ∎ ∎

CHAPTER SIX

ASCENDING

"Triumph is the 'umph' added to try."
Anonymous

My cousin Sydney—I am the oldest of 18 cousins on my mother's side, and Sydney is the youngest–made a brightly colored rainbow drawing that hung on the ceiling above my bed in Santa Clara. I remember focusing on it, and now I like to say that her drawing gave me hope for brighter days ahead. I imagined her coloring it and thinking of cheering up her oldest cousin living in the hospital for five months. My father thought it worth noting that, on the 25th of May, 2004, I actually looked at the rainbow on command.

Ten days after I had begun plunging into another abyss thanks to increasing pressure on my brain, my temperature was normal, my white blood cell count unchanging, my liver enzyme improving, and my left arm splint taken off. My range of movement was improving slightly, and physical therapists were back on the job. My doctor ordered an EEG in my coma state. Things felt dark, but my body was still pushing quietly behind my blank stare.

On the last day of May, I blinked "yes" twice for my brother and began to track my eyes to sight as well as sound. The fingers on my right hand were still tightly gnarled, and I couldn't extend them without pain—at least my parents assumed the grimaces on my face meant pain. My shoulders and elbows had a range of movement of 90 degrees, my wrist 80 degrees. Most important, though, I smiled deliberately at

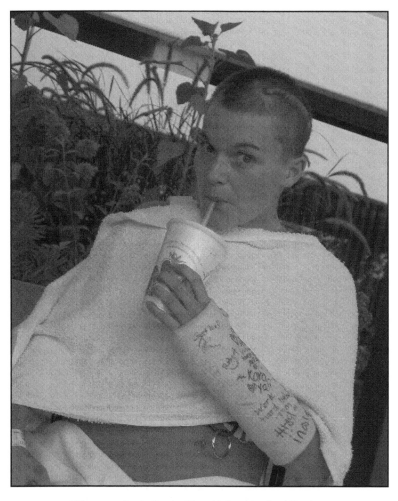

Still recovering in Santa Clara Valley Medical Center.

my Grammy and friend Heidi. May was over, and maybe the worst with it.

During the first week in June, nearly two months after the accident, my tracking of people moving was finally improving again. I began to smile a few times a day, though an old cap on my front tooth had come off in the accident, and my family found that snaggletooth look curiously disconcerting. In the face of everything else, it seemed so small, but it was one more indignity. Around this time I looked at myself in the mirror and reportedly smiled—I must have been in a sorry state to smile at my raggedy mouth, my shaved head, and hollow cheeks.

On June 9th, the shunt in my head was cleaned and replaced. Looking back, this seems to be the truly big turning point. The shunt was finally working properly—relieving pressure—and it wasn't infected, relieving me of two major battle fronts.

Therapists began to push me to sit up. Two months after being hit, I could sit at a 45-degree angle, with a goal of 90 degrees by the next day. I was still wearing a neck collar, but that came off early in June. In the middle of June, I was able to eat a few small ice chips with my therapists–a big step toward eating solid food. I was shown books, and it looked to my family as if I were moving my eyes left to right in response to seeing the words. A few days after that, I actually read basic commands like "Look at Dad," "Look at the ceiling," "Look at TV, feet, rainbow . . ." I really could read. A VERY GOOD DAY, my dad wrote in big capitals and put the words in a box in his journal entry for June 13th. He also thought I showed unusual interest in the tasks at which I now would have to work to achieve: "She likes to look at her hand," he wrote, "as she works on strengthening it." I am an athlete, and I was responding like an athlete to a bigger challenge than I'd ever faced.

My cousins and friends came to visit, and my parents liked seeing me perk up a bit with them. Maybe the biggest relief was that my sense of humor hadn't been destroyed. Long before I could speak or do much else, my cousin Cory asked me if I were hungry. I nodded. Cory asked if I were so hungry I could eat my arm. I lifted my left arm to my chin and opened my mouth, grinning as best I could. Everyone laughed, so I did it again.

First, though, I had to sit up—and balance, too. Then I had to eat and drink on my own. Then I had to learn to transfer to a wheelchair. Then I had to move the wheelchair. Then I had to get out of the wheelchair. Talking would help. And I had to do everything better, include remember. These tasks would take months, up to years, to accomplish.

A little more than a week after my VERY GOOD DAY, I finally began to communicate verbally. My mom and brother were on the phone with my dad, and they put the phone up to my ear so that my dad could talk to me. These were not two-way conversations up to this point. Much to their surprise, I took a deep breath and mouthed the words "Hi, Dad." After some encouragement, I attempted it again. The third time I managed to produce a barely audible squeak–to which my family responded with overwhelming excitement. Within a few days, by June 25, I was using four-to-five word sentences. With this, however, came the realization of the extent of my brain injury.

At first, my only communication consisted of things like "yes," "no," and "more." As time wore on and my awareness increased, however, my communication became more complex and at times difficult for my family. Whenever they would leave the room, I would get upset and squeak "Take me with you!" or "Don't leave me here," or "I want to go home." And, upon my re-discovering of my voice, I would tell lies when I could not remember the real answer. My brother would listen to these preposterous answers and say, "Really?" Then, I'd laugh, realizing I totally just made up an answer. My friend Becky would ask me what I did that day, expecting to hear about some therapy, but instead I would tell her, "Oh, I walked around on the roof" or "I ate salami and cheese," even though I was getting my nutrition through a feeding tube until July.

I remember it being a milestone for me to answer the phone or use the nurse's call button by my bed. Within a week of my first words, I grew to love the phone. Even though I mangled some words and concepts, I was understandable. I even answered the phone myself every so often.

Yet things didn't continue to go in one direction. I was still confused. Just after I began talking in late June, I convinced the nurses at SCVMC that I absolutely had to call my parents, and I couldn't wait another minute. I thought

I was in Colfax, near my parents' house, and I couldn't understand why I was stuck there. The nurses were alarmed by my agitation, so they let me call my parents. I proceeded to explain to them that I had been in a bad accident and that they would need to come pick me up as soon as possible. They patiently explained that I was in Santa Clara, which is about three hours from Colfax. I was actually thinking about the hill on Meadow Drive and thought that I just got the town name wrong. Brains are so weird. I shouted into the phone, "Just come pick me up!"

My family was used to my begging to be permitted go home with them. One night, though, I kept insisting that I wanted to sleep "back there," pointing to a big closet in my hospital room. My brother opened the door for me—making it clear that I'd been asking to sleep in the closet. "Aren't you going to put me to bed?" I asked. Seeing the closet, though, I felt silly—and Dan felt worried. My brain injury moved me in so many unpredictable ways.

Daniel and Danh came to visit me one Friday after a strenuous bike ride. I was glad Daniel hadn't quit riding, and I was glad that they had become fast friends and riding buddies while I was languishing in the hospital. Anyway, they looked around for the food always plentiful in my hospital room, gifts from friends. They started stuffing bundt cake in their mouths and were startled when I said, peevishly, "Hey! Give me some of that!" The men were shocked by the loudness of my voice, its clarity, and my persistence.

I had not yet eaten any solid food aside from ice chips

under the careful supervision of my therapists. You can imagine how desperate I must have been to taste real food. Dan was extremely nervous that I'd choke on it, but I got Danh on my side, and we didn't let up until Dan agreed that I could have some. He ran a test case by putting the smallest bit in his mouth to see if it would dissolve–and it did. After explaining that I would just put it on my tongue and let it dissolve, he gave me a little piece. I did not hesitate a moment and immediately scarfed it down. He said the happy look on my face was priceless. After that, I convinced him to give me some more! I wish I could remember the exquisite joy of tasting food after three months. I must have been in heaven. Shortly after that, I was able to eat all of my meals by mouth again.

Just before my 27th birthday on July 9, some friends and family came to SCVMC to celebrate with me. After eating a little cheesecake from my friend Nicole a day earlier, I must have dislodged another tooth that had been cracked in the accident. I felt something in my mouth, and, as I was opening presents, complained loudly that we had to do something "about this gum problem." Everyone tried to distract me— she's not herself, after all, and she can't possibly have gum, no one gave her any, and let's just talk about something else. I wouldn't let it rest, though, and finally Daniel told me to spit it out. What came out wasn't gum but my tooth, an unpleasant birthday event, but I remember being delighted they finally believed me. We think my molar must have been cracked in the accident but hadn't been disturbed since by chewing.

As I improved, I could wheel myself in my chair from my room to the deck at SCVMC. The distance was probably only 100 yards, from my room, past the nurses' station, through the hallway, through the dining room, and to the deck. I was very proud of myself for this accomplishment. I was given botox shots in my right arm to ease tone, and that helped my strength and agility. On July 10th, a deep vein thrombosis was discovered in my right groin, and the doctors inserted an umbrella filter. It didn't seem to interfere with my progress.

Because I was in the hospital for so long, I made a lot of friends among the patients and nurses. One friend, Julie, was not paralyzed but had a more serious head injury than mine that forced her to have to re-learn how to walk. Driving in the early morning darkness to work with the cows at California State Polytechnic University, she swerved to avoid hitting a deer and crashed her car. Apparently, she was stuck in her car for a few hours, and the paramedics had to use the Jaws of Life to pry her out of the car. The lack of oxygen to her brain caused her weakness. When therapists stretched her too hard, she would "yell" in an intense whisper, "It hurts so bad, I'm going to scream!" Another friend, Jared, was also in a car accident. He was a high school senior, and his dad was a battalion chief with the Kern County Fire Department. Jared was not talking in the hospital yet, so he used "yes" and "no" buttons to communicate. After he was released from the hospital, he was able to go to the senior ball with one of his friends.

My therapists were also good to me: Jennifer, Theresa, Erin, Vicki, Ron, Benny, and Scott. Theresa later attended one of my presentations at San Jose's Presentation High School in December 2006. She was an alumna of the school, something I didn't know at the time. While I was in the hospital, she took me to the cafeteria for a special "field trip" to select my lunch—which got me out of the routine hospital-served lunch. Scott, the recreational therapist, took us to eat sushi, to a Los Gatos Picnic in the Park, to Beppo's, and he took me swimming in the SCVMC pool during the rare times I did not have a bladder infection, something quite common with spinal cord injured-patients. (Now I am on a prophylactic medication that I take every day to ward off these infections.)

A few of the nurses became my friends as well: Mary Lou and Mary Ann, the nurse manager. Mary Lou had a certain way of talking with a cute accent that I miss hearing! She really watched over me in the hospital and made sure I had everything I needed in her systematic way.

There were, however, a few nurses who got it all wrong. My family and I called them the C or D team; whereas the best group was the A team. One crushed my pills and put them in applesauce and contacted my parents when I would not take my pills. Smartly, my mom reminded them that it said in bold print on my chart, "Takes her pills whole with a liquid.

NO APPLESAUCE!" Imagine the taste of the applesauce with mashed pills in it!

Sounds became part of my daily ritual. Each of us had a nurse's call button to use—part of my therapy had been to learn to use the button and to ask for help when I needed it. "Bing! Bing! Bing!" We heard all day long from the other rooms (and mine). Three times a day, we heard the clanging of the food trays, delivering dishes that I remember as largely boring or tasteless. The most difficult sound, though, was the terrible bleating coming from the room down the hall of an especially bad brain injury patient. We felt really sad for him and his family.

As I got stronger, I'd push myself out to the deck, and we'd often have lunch at the table in the sunshine. My parents made me use my right hand for at least a few bites in the meal. A few days after my birthday on July 9th, I was using a spoon and a fork, but I hated having to use my bad arm. July 23rd was my first outing to Bucca di Beppo's restaurant in a van with the other patients. I couldn't stand how people were looking at me. Alan's mother Rita joined us at this dinner and, at this point, I still was not quite sure who she was. I smiled and was polite, but it was not until just before bed that night that my parents had to remind me who she was.

On July 27th, I sent an email to my brother and mom and dad using my left index finger—I even remembered their email addresses. I didn't remember Alan's email address, though, and still really didn't remember him. In August I was reading an email from my alma mater, Santa Clara University, when I stumbled across an announcement of a service at the mission for my injuries and Alan's death. I'd been ready for a mid-day therapy session when I read the announcement, but I remember asking about him. My parents showed me a picture of us together in December 2003. I do not remember feeling sad about it at first, but I do remember feeling a deep sense of loss like a strong undercurrent that would not reveal itself for at least a year. I'm sure it must have been difficult for them to have to repeat themselves so much about his death just as it was hard for me to have to continuously re-learn of his loss.

Throughout August, I gained a little needed weight and pushed myself further in my wheelchair. The nurses used to weigh my chair and then weigh me in it to keep track of how much weight I had gained. Best of all, I was back on a perfectly ordinary diet, which meant I could eat things like chocolate, nuts, and dairy foods. This would help me gain some weight back. Now I could eat all of the forbidden foods pictured on the terrible poster in my room that my cousin Matthew said when he looked at it: "Looks good!" By early September, I was nearly ready to go home, but the hospital insisted I needed some practice. With that good news, I also got a free pass to go to Grammy's house in San Rafael for the day. I even contributed to Dan's daily updating of my website that day: "Thank you for everything during this hard time," I made him write, "and thanks to my parents and brother for everything. I love you guys!" It wasn't eloquent, but it was important.

My trip to Grammy's was mostly memorable because of the food. I didn't talk much because I was busy eating and my brain was still in a fog. Miss Social was not interacting with anyone or anything but the appetizers. It was a huge thing for my family, and it was even great for me seeing the world again after being cooped up for so long. I remember the catheterization thing was an issue because my mom had only done it a few times with nurses watching her do it. My aunt Paula, a nurse, helped her as I laid on Grammy's bed, so tired I took a nap! We drove back to SCVMC along the ocean in San Francisco, but I was too busy taking another cat nap on the way back to the hospital to look at it again. I remember not wanting to go back to the hospital, but we did.

We used another off-site pass to go to Santa Cruz to see my friend Sarah. The beach-side restaurant was packed, and it was a sunny day so our table was partly outside. After lunch, the four of us went out on the Santa Cruz pier and watched the Pacific ocean. Sarah started playing with my hair, and the combination of that with the afternoon sun made me close my eyes and become very relaxed! I think I probably took a little cat nap–a common occurrence in the early days of my injury.

A night or two before I was discharged, we stayed in a house just off the hospital grounds. We had to prove we could manage an ordinary setting. We did. A group of friends came to visit me from the Mountain View Masters Swim Team, and they brought me dinner. Much as I wanted to enjoy the normal food, I wasn't able to each much because my eating pace had really slowed down and I was anxious to see many of my friends. My friends Danh, Mariska, their son Tyler, and Erin all came to see me as well. Tyler had been born to Danh and Mariska the end of July, so he was still a newborn. Then I went home, not to the little Cupertino apartment nearby that I had shared with my cat Charlie, but back to Grass Valley.

▪ ▪ ▪

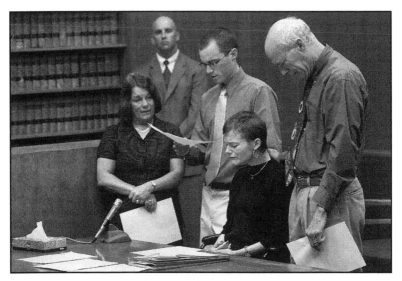

Mason family at Harvey Hereford's trial September 27, 2004.
Reprinted with permission of Christopher Chung and the Santa Rosa
Press Democrat

CHAPTER SEVEN

Sentencing Harvey Hereford to San Quentin Prison

" . . . it is sometimes hard to forget the fact that this was not just an accident. "

Daniel Mason

The sentencing for Harvey Hereford was originally scheduled for July 2004, when I was still in the hospital, but the assistant district attorney convinced the judge to move the sentencing until a time when I could attend because they thought my presence would be important for the judge to see. Within a couple of weeks after I went home to Grass Valley, we headed to Santa Rosa and the court. My Uncle Mark got us two rooms at a Petaluma hotel about fifteen minutes from the courthouse. We had a great dinner that night at a restaurant recommended by my aunt Sue and uncle Brian, and, oddly, it was the first time I felt like a non-paralyzed person simply going out to eat with my family.

After charges were filed against him following the accident in April, Harvey Hereford waived a preliminary hearing and eventually pleaded guilty to manslaughter and driving under the influence, causing serious bodily injury. His blood alcohol level was reported to be more than three times the legal limit. Unfortunately, the district attorney couldn't find enough evidence to charge him with second-degree murder because they couldn't prove intent. Hereford's attorney agreed to a five-year enhancement because of the death of Alan and the nature of my injuries.

Mark, the lawyer of the family, told us that at the sentencing we would have a chance to speak before the judge, Elaine Rushing (who happened to be a cyclist), gave the sentence. In a case like this, though, he warned us that the judge wouldn't have much discretion.

My dad kept notes at the sentencing. "The courtroom

was filled with Alan's and Jill's friends, bike coalition members, and family," he wrote. "All four of us testified to the judge and Harvey. Jill's speech was the most powerful and moving. None of us were sure we could speak, but we all did. Alan's maternal grandmother gave Harvey a good tongue-lashing. This was a beginning for us and a beginning of closure for the Lius."

Here's part of what my dad said: "Until Jill was hit by Mr. Hereford, she lived life to its fullest. She loved life and people, and everyone fortunate enough to meet Jill never forgot her. Family and friends were so important to her that she would do anything for any one of them. She possessed boundless energy and approached everything with great enthusiasm and excitement.

"Speaking as a father and husband, I am saddened to see how this tragedy is affecting our family. My wife is burdened by the pressures of morning, afternoon, evening, and night responsibilities, leaving little or no time for herself. My son is sacrificing his most productive years due to his love of Jill. In my children's adult life, Jill has been Dan's best friend as they biked or ran several times a week, participated in triathlons together, and spent at least one night a week together cooking, eating, and sharing new stories about their lives.

"He now devotes hours weekly updating the website about Jill's progress and spending numerous weekends with the family, instead of doing what most 24-year-olds would do. Do not get me wrong; Daniel, being such a devoted brother, is not complaining, yet I do worry. He even gave up biking for several months. As for myself, I am burdened with constant concern for Jill, Dan, and Mom; and I know that my most perfect daughter has changed forever. Life will get better, but it will be different."

My mom made Harvey listen to the details of the wonderful ordinariness of our lives, all now changed: "On Friday, April 9, we had dinner in Pleasanton for Larry's birthday. Dan had a bike race the next day so the rest of us drove to Cupertino to stay at Jill's apartment. After breakfast on Saturday we did some preliminary research because Jill wanted to buy a condominium.

"Then we all headed to Grammy's in Marin for an early Easter celebration. Alan wasn't with us because he had a swim meet. We did have a grand time with aunts, uncles, and cousins. On Sunday morning, Jill woke each of us to say goodbye before she left to meet Alan in Santa Rosa for a training ride and Easter dinner with his family.

"We spent a quiet Sunday with Grammy and then headed back to Grass Valley. Before we reached Highway 37, we received the telephone call that shattered our lives: Jill had been hit while riding her bike and had severe head and back injuries.

"It is impossible to list all of the losses Jill will have as the result of being hit by Mr. Hereford on that Easter Sunday. She was an avid runner and triathlete. She had a full life in which she balanced work, social life, training, and family relationships. She had a relationship with Alan that made her very happy.

"Her severe closed brain injury resulted in a coma. She has hydrocephalous and has a permanent ventricular-peritoneal shunt. She still has difficulties with memory, logic, and other cognitive functions. Jill was unable to speak until the end of June. In July she began eating food instead of getting her nutrition from a feeding tube in her stomach. Her shoulders are very stiff and inhibit movement of both her arms. Her right arm has lasting neurological damage but is beginning to move five months after the injury. She is now paralyzed and will most likely be in a wheelchair for the rest of her life.

"Jill moved back home with us when she was discharged from the rehab center. We hired someone to help with Jill's care while we are at work. When we can, we will try to bring Jill back to the Santa Clara area to visit friends and old co-workers. Jill's life will be very different from what she hoped for: continue her career in marketing, buy a place, maybe settle down with someone, have a family in a few years, continue to travel, do triathlons, keep in touch with EVERYONE.

"While we try to have hope and are extremely grateful that Jill's life was spared, it is very sad to think of how much she has lost. There is nothing the court can do to give Jill back the life that she once had, but we hope that people will take note of our family's loss and think about its root cause in one individual's failure to make responsible choices."

My brother Daniel talked about the impact on our parents especially: "We've heard just a little bit about how much Alan and Jill have lost as a result of this devastating accident. But it is also important to remember that in addition to the loss of Alan's life and the devastating injuries that Jill has suffered, there have been many other lives impacted by this tragic event. In Jill's case, for example, our parents have shouldered the largest share of the load.

"After spending five months of their lives at Jill's bedside in the hospital, they have brought Jill back into their house and have made caring for her their single highest priority in life. They don't have the time or the energy for anything else. They have literally dropped everything from their previous life. My parents are tough, and they will persevere, but I have watched them age what seems like 20 years in the last five months. This crime has taken an immeasurable toll on them. . .

"Such a diverse and widespread group of people came to bring their encouragement. Even the website that Jill's work friends set up for her after the accident has become quite a popular internet destination. The amazing thing is the site still gets over 250 hits per day from people checking for updates about her progress. Even more amazing is that the site has been viewed over 50,000 times since her accident.

"Jill has come a long way since her first few weeks clinging to life in the ICU just five months ago. She has opened her eyes, she has smiled, she has even learned to eat and speak again. I am extremely grateful to be able to just sit and talk with my sister again. The progress that she has shown is nothing short of miraculous.

"But despite all of the progress, this tragedy will change Jill's life forever. Jill worked very hard to get to where she was before the accident and so much of that was just taken away from her in an instant. She will work hard again but towards very different goals.

"The most terrifying part about it is that this whole chain of events was brought on by the irresponsible and 100% preventable actions of one single human. I don't have the energy to really be angry at Mr. Hereford, but it is sometimes hard to forget the fact that this was not just an accident."

While the court was packed with family and friends of Alan and me, from what we could tell, no one was there for Harvey. Hereford's lawyer requested another judge because he thought the one assigned to the case was too hard on criminals, but the new one happened to be a cyclist. The judge cried during a DVD shown during the trial that depicted how active Alan had been.

Hereford addressed the court. But when he asked if the family had questions, the judge said, "I don't think that's a good idea," and shook her head to say no. She ended up giving him the maximum sentence– which was only 8 years and a few months, pitiful for killing someone and totally changing another's life. The reason for this short sentence is infuriating: there was no INTENT to kill because Hereford was too drunk. Since then, the jail sent me a letter saying Hereford would be released early on "good behavior." What I want to know is how you are "bad" in prison? I think some laws need to be changed. So, he will be free in 2012, I'll be forever in a wheelchair, and Alan is never coming home.

After the hearing, I was interviewed just outside the courtroom by several local newspapers. I was overwhelmed by friends and family who came to the trial. Many people from my mom's side of the family went to lunch. We sat at a long table at the restaurant and Alan's family and some of his friends were there, too.

■   ■   ■

PART TWO: LIFE BEGINS

CHAPTER EIGHT

ARRIVING HOME: CHILDHOOD REVISITED

"Muddy water, let stand, becomes clear."

Lao Tzu

From the time I was injured in April until I was released from Santa Clara Valley Medical Center in September, my parents spent every free moment with me in the hospital. At the same time, they had to cope with what I had left behind: an apartment, a car, a cat, and with what I would have to face in the future. They simply ignored what they had left behind in Grass Valley as best they could.

The first priority was my immediate medical care, but even from the first day after the accident they had to deal with insurance and money. Because I am an independent adult, they could not decide for me or act in my name. My parents simply had to do their best with no legal authority. When Dr. Duong determined that I could make my own decisions, it was a time for hope. My uncle had set a hearing date for a conservatorship, but I had improved, and Dr. Duong would not sign the court papers that would have declared me incapable of managing my own affairs.

Once it was settled that I would be going back to Grass Valley and not to my own apartment, my parents were able to cancel the lease on my apartment. My apartment happened to be near the hospital and so it had been something of a godsend in giving them a place to stay that was familiar. It was an expensive godsend, however, and had to be cut loose. With heavy hearts, my family stored all my things, some at a storage place in Grass Valley, some in their house, and some in an uncle's work warehouse. It felt like a death of sorts— they had no idea if and when I'd see my things again. The family came together with trucks and busy hands to move me out.

Then, they turned to what I'd need in the house itself. My childhood home is a rambler at the end of a winding road, set back in the woods around Grass Valley, a foothill town on the way to Lake Tahoe. A two-and-a-half-car garage is attached, with two steps to climb to the back door. The front door has a step up to a slab and another step to get inside. Once in, there's another step down to the living room. Steps we had never noticed suddenly loomed large as hurdles.

My girlhood bedroom was filled with a large double

bed into which I could no longer climb. The hall bathroom, recently beautifully renovated, had a door so narrow I couldn't get in, and once in, I couldn't turn my chair or transfer to the toilet.

Two of my uncles and some family friends seized the initiative in making the house accessible, not an easy thing to do either in the seizing or the doing. They installed a ramp in the garage so I could get in the door from the garage to the laundry room and do my transferring from the car to the chair out of the rain and snow. They cut out the cabinet under the bathroom sink so I could roll under it. They remounted the door on offset hinges so I could get into the bathroom; they removed the closet to enlarge the bathroom and make another door. Friends gave us portable ramps to use for the living room and the deck so I could roll my chair down and sit by the wood stove or go out and enjoy the sun.

At the same time, family and friends had to re-think access to their houses and bathroom arrangements in anticipation and hope that I'd be able to visit. Two uncles installed a metal bar in their bathroom so I could use the bathroom more easily when I visit them, and another made extra transfer boards to keep at all my relatives' houses. One of my aunts rigged up a good temporary solution for me to manage her tiny bathroom—a big curtain that closes off the hall when the door is taken off its hinges. When they bought a new house, her husband got offset hinges for the bathroom door, moved the toilet, and cut off the bottom of the door frame so I could wheel into the bathroom. My brother's apartment in San Francisco has been the toughest: he lives up a lot of stairs with no elevator. I hate it that he has to carry me, but I'd hate more not to visit.

The entire time of my hospitalization from April through September, neighbors, friends, and workmates watched my parents' house, brought in mail, raked leaves, and cut down branches and trees. My mom's Union Hill School friends and our closest neighbors made countless meals for us, scheduling nights that stretched into six months after I got home. Grammy came to stay through October and November, taking a lot of pressure off my parents as they eased back to work in a new school year and, far tougher, suddenly had to take care of someone long gone from home and now utterly dependent on them.

My friend Becky flew home from San Diego to Santa Rosa the night after the accident. Her family offered a house in Santa Rosa for my parents to stay in for the next few weeks. Later she wrote to me that she would never forget the image of her dad walking with my dad to the car. "He looked like a broken man... so emotionally drained, he could barely walk." Children know "how much our parents love us," she wrote, "but seeing your dad like that was a physical sign to me of just how much they love us."

Both my parents, my brother and my extended family aged terribly that first year. They soldiered on impressively, and they've regained their incredible strength and resilience. I cannot say often enough, though, how meaningful the support from family and friends—and many, many people

I will never know—was to me and to my parents and brother. We could not have managed without it.

Not long after I returned to Grass Valley, many friends held an auction/karaoke night for me at the Holiday Cabaret, a bar in downtown Grass Valley. People donated things to auction, including a road bike. Many of my old teachers and a number of old friends were there. A few people sang, and I thought they would want to hear me sing. However, my singing voice did not make a showing that evening. It had only been a few months since any semblance of my speaking voice had even made a showing, and I had only been out of the hospital for a short time. I now mostly only sing quietly to myself because I know what a singer I used to be at weddings and funerals. I have no head voice like I used to have, which is very frustrating. I can still sight-read music, but reaching those higher notes is ugly.

My dad kept a journal in the first few months I was home, wanting to be sure to note my progress. According to his journal, six months after the accident, I still required full assistance with transfers, couldn't sit without support and took one or two naps a day. My caregiver Christy said my mother told her not to leave my side when I was sitting on the bed. My conversation was minimal—I only responded in my very soft voice that rose a little for phone conversations, but otherwise was barely heard. I said the same things three-to-five times in a few hours and had a terrible time with my short-term memory.

Fairly soon after getting home, I could push my chair

on a bare floor—my left arm was gaining some strength—but only about five inches on the carpet. I started transferring from the chair to bed, and vice versa, with a transfer board, an ordeal that would take about twenty minutes. I wouldn't position the board or take it out. I can still see Christy sitting on the floor leaning against the wall drinking coffee as I struggled to transfer. After about a month, though, I cut the transfer time to ten minutes. Transferring from the car into my chair was even harder. I remember the incredible pride I felt when I transferred from Christy's car on my own for the first time in the Long's parking lot in Grass Valley.

In the hospital they had given me some botox for my gnarled right hand that I kept folded to my chest. Because of the head injury, my right upper extremity continues to be numb. I had a therapist tell me smartly: "You are a triplegic!" The botox in my bicep helped ease the tightness, but only after a number of shots. I can't believe people get this shot voluntarily—it's administered with a huge six-inch needle and is very painful. The first didn't work, and neither did the second or third. Apparently the nerve to inject is hard to find. They keep stabbing until they find the right nerve. This was consciously the first time I had felt pain.

After the series of shots, though, my right arm did relax, although I could only raise it to chest level. I can still only raise it to my shoulder. I worked hard on trying to use my right hand. I couldn't extend my right fingers, and my thumb wouldn't budge even with my dad's help. At first, I only used my left hand on the keyboard for email and starting this book, but then, out of necessity, I pushed myself to use it for eating, brushing my teeth with an electric toothbrush, drying my hair, pushing my chair and getting dressed. In the hospital, my family made a rule that I take at least two bites with my right hand during every meal.

Still, I let my right thumb "cheat" when I push my chair. I used to have extra spaces on the push rings of the wheels on the right side of my chair to allow my thumb to fall in and use the bars that hold the ring as leverage to propel my chair. Now, I simply grab the entire wheel with my right hand, which makes my hand dirty, but it's much easier now that either wheel works, especially when I put my chair together getting out of my car.

■　■　■

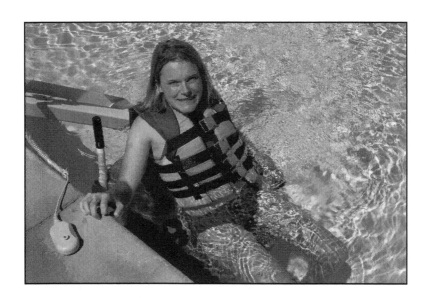

CHAPTER NINE

THERAPIES: SLOW BUT SURE

*"Whenever you are asked if you can do a job, tell 'em,
'Certainly, I can!' Then get busy and find out how to do it."*
Theodore Roosevelt

The first order of business after I returned to Grass
Valley was finding someone to take care of me while my
parents worked. We needed highly specialized at-home care
and worked through an agency to find it. The first caregiver
who turned up fell asleep for a lot of the day, and the second
couldn't drive me anywhere for one reason or another. The

third was fired by me after my jewelry disappeared. Like a small child, I was easy to take advantage of—I couldn't remember much and certainly couldn't get around fast enough to see what they were doing. I also was taking two or three naps every day, so they had plenty of time for their shenanigans.

My mother also left elaborate directions for the caregivers so they would know what I needed to accomplish. I certainly wasn't going to remember the routine. It's strange for me now to read her list because it shows how bad my head injury was. Here are some of the things she wanted me to do:

Shift weight at least every hour (we set a timer)

Elevate legs when possible

Watch fluid intake-about 1,800-2,000 cc's/day (1oz. = 30 cc)

4 oz. juice @ breakfast + 8 oz. Citrucel

8 oz. juice/water lunch

2 8 oz. water/juice between lunch & dinner

2 8 oz. water dinner & after

Practice writing left and right handed

Do exercises under home program in Rehab Binder

Range legs

Practice lifting, stretching, etc. with right arm/hand

Read binders on Traumatic Brain Injury and Spinal Cord Injury

Check emails/website

Call friends

My mom came home every day at lunch to catheterize me—I couldn't do it myself and didn't want anyone else to do it. Poor Mom. Grammy was here then but was unable to transfer me.

Catheterization is how most spinal cord-injured people pee. Basically, I insert a catheter (a small tube) into my bladder to drain the urine. It is different with every injury, but I figure out when I need to go based on the clock and how much liquid I have ingested. In my case, I also I have a neurogenic bladder (part of the head injury) which turns out to be a plus because I am prescribed one catheter each time I go to the bathroom. A few times, when the company has needed proof that I "still have a neurogenic bladder and cannot pee without a catheter," I have had to wait for the necessary paperwork to be faxed from my doctor to the catheter company, proving that "yes, my condition is unchanging." It is very frustrating because it is like a slap in the face every year it happens. "Oh, you can't pee on your own yet? We're sorry, we'll just take a month or so to get you the supplies you need once we get the proof from your doctor—every year."

My parents probably despaired as we lurched from one bad caregiver to another. In December, some three months after I was back in Grass Valley, the same agency sent us Christy. When people say that there are always some good parts mixed in with tragedy, Christy comes to mind. She stayed with me for two full years, even after I eventually moved to Sacramento, and we are good friends now.

We had a lot in common in the sense of shared interests

and sudden losses. A level-10 gymnast, Christy earned a full scholarship to California Polytechnic in San Luis Obispo, but she got pregnant before she could get to school. She has raised Dylan, a joy of a boy, on her own. I think her own courage and her focus on Dylan has been good for me to see. She never gives up trying to make the life she's living better.

I couldn't be left alone at all–we also had to hire a service to provide at-home therapy. Rehab without Walls, a company identified by Aetna, my employer's insurance company, helped me with the transition from hospital to outpatient rehabilitation. All therapists—speech, occupational, physical, and psychological—came to my parents' house, and I did not have to go anywhere too often right away. One of the hardest things I remember having to do was wheel down the hallway in my clunky wheelchair and transfer into bed. Getting in and out of the car was a lot harder: out the door, down the steep ramp, twenty minutes to transfer in, my parents disassembling the chair.

Beginning in January 2005, three months after I returned to Grass Valley, I had to go to the local hospital for therapy. I was so out of it then, a rolling zombie. No talking, almost no facial expressions. Even though most of those months are lost to me, I do remember my therapists' excitement in the spring of 2005 when I was introduced to the "Widget Guy" who had developed a lever-driven chair. I decided to roll up the driveway so I could try the widget on the downhill. When I think of it now, I wonder at their excitement, but I think I wasn't showing a lot of initiative or interest. They also pushed me to work on going up and down curbs, something I still cannot do.

By February 2005, I ate my first right-handed meal and started using my right hand on the computer keyboard and for writing in my log. I remembered Daniel's cell telephone number, and I went down the steep garage ramp with minimal assistance. Once, though, as I was rolling down the ramp into the garage with Christy watching, I got into a laughing fit and slammed into the dresser at the bottom of the ramp!

By March 2005, I could sit on the floor, with help getting down and back up, of course. I managed the garage ramp without any help at all and could get nearly a quarter of the way back up the slope. I could transfer from the therapy mattress to the chair without a board. Using a stopwatch, my dad kept track of my "driveway time trials" and my speeds consistently improved. I would time myself wheeling the length of the driveway. My brother Dan's coaching rolled through my head as I pushed faster and faster: Don't lean, don't laugh, don't look at it, thumb straight! I played the piano (not well) with both hands and read the music.

Early on, Dan made me memorize the name of his riding team. As I got better, we moved on to the names of his master's degree classes in mechanical engineering at Stanford. Mechanics! Feedback Control Design! Situation Failure Analysis! None of it easy, but I needed the push to make my memory work.

By April 2005, a year after the accident, I finally started

caring how I looked. I wore my first skirt and heels and spoke on the telephone for thirty minutes! My parents and brother helped me dress and undress, so it was a milestone when I could do it myself. I remember working on this "skill" in therapy on the mat with big hospital scrubs, of course bigger than probably two pairs of my own pants. I had tried dressing on my bed but realized it was much easier in my chair, especially after showering, because for me, it's almost impossible to transfer to bed with a wet fanny. I use various tools, like a dressing stick, a reacher, an a long-handled shoe horn. My short-term memory began to improve, and I started to remember where I'd left things. I found my electronic calendar and deleted recurring events that, sadly, would no longer recur: runs, swims, and triathlons.

I got faster with the whole peeing process. I stopped peeing from the bed and started to pee with the chair next to the toilet. The first time I ICPed in the toilet was in a Davis gas station bathroom. I had a mirror to put between my legs so I could get "a hole in one" as Christy used to say. When I went to my ten-year high school reunion, I had to use the mirror before we left, but thankfully didn't need it at the reunion because there was no way I was carting that thing with me.

In May 2005, I submerged my head in the pool, something I am hugely reluctant to do. I took fifteen steps with a walker during therapy using my hip flexors. I needed NO help peeing at least four times. Once, when my mom came home from work at the end of the day, she said "Okay, it's time to pee." As if I were following her train of thought, I started rolling back to my bedroom. where I was catheterized in the first months at home. And then, I said, "I already did!" Imagine the excitement when she realized that this time constraint was off her shoulders.

By September 2005, I could complete the catheterization without a mirror. I remembered all eight restaurants to which Christy and I had gone to in Grass Valley. I could transfer from bed to chair and chair to bed in less than three minutes, and I could do five-to-ten full-wheel push-ups, which are very important for pressure relief. I started to read the newspaper and to be able to refer to the articles in conversation, which my dad was thrilled about. I absolutely began to rely on my Palm Pilot and was able to do some of the website updates. I sang "Happy Birthday" to my mother, which meant a lot to them, but my voice wasn't much and not even close to what it used to be. I started to chew gum (And it actually wasn't a broken tooth like in the hospital)!

About this time, I started thinking about moving to Sacramento, a decision I finally made based on my upcoming therapies at University of California (UC) Davis Med Center and my need to once again move away from home (Hadn't I already done that?). I remember the day I went into my therapy at Sierra Nevada Memorial Hospital, absolutely sure about my move to Sacramento. My therapists noticed that once my mind was made up, that was it. My "sass," as my counselor Emily put it, was back to stay.

The problem was where I would live in Sacramento. I

needed to find a place that would fit me and my wheelchair. Over the course of a few days, my parents painstakingly drove me around to 20 different apartment complexes. First they would get out to check out the complex, knowing just what I needed. If it passed their initial approval, I would transfer out of the car and check it out myself. This was very sweet, and something I think many parents would not think of, but mine did! We looked at a few I remember: one was in an area close to where I ended up living. It had large hallways, which is a must for a wheelchair. One we looked at had an indentation in the door, as if someone had gotten upset and punched a hole in the door. I wouldn't be living there anyway because I couldn't fit in the bathroom.

In August 2006, I finally moved out of my parents' home, even though I was still so out of it. We chose a new apartment complex in the South area of Sacramento. One of my former lacrosse teammate's co-workers was my roommate, and we were two of the first tenants. When we moved in, they were still constructing several of the other apartment buildings. The apartment that was slated for us was not completed yet, so we moved into a temporary apartment for two months. Turns out, the apartment they were going to move us into was rented to someone else, so they put us in another unit, which happened to be a little pricier and overlooked the pool and putting green and was on the ground floor. The pool even had a lift, although I confess I didn't use the pool more than a couple of times in two years because it was a long process to get a suit on, then wheel back to my apartment wet and eventually cold, get in the shower and change.

I hired Christy for a few months to come to my place in Sacramento, instead of Grass Valley, from her home in Auburn in order to drive me places and just to be with me in what was a scary move and the transition. Prior to my Grandmother Mason giving me my home Internet access, I remember forgetting where the computer room was in my apartment complex and having to ask the office staff to show me where it was located. Just writing that makes me realize how messed up my brain was. I lived in the apartment for two years, growing very used to my routines of calling for the bus, doing therapy at UC Davis Med Center, going to the Spinal Cord Injury support group at UCD, and taking driving lessons for about six months.

One of my UC Davis physical therapists connected me with his former graduate school physical therapy professor form Sacramento State. I have since been volunteering for the practical portion of the course and have had four groups of PT students use me as their "patient." Groups have done so much for me: they've figured out a great exercise program for arm strengthening, getting off the floor, transferring into the car and stowing my chair, writing with my affected right hand, and transferring techniques. When I participate, I go to Sac State every Friday during their class semesters and do their practical final exam with them. It is great for me because I can teach new physical therapists what works for a real person as opposed what they may read in a textbook. And I always enjoy meeting new people!

I also worked hard with physical, occupational and speech therapists from the UC Davis Med Center in Sacramento. They showed me weights to use to strengthen my arms, an effort that continues to be important. They also helped show me the best ways to get off the floor and into my chair, which I still (five plus years later) cannot do. Only once have I been able to get from the floor into my chair. I was transferring from my chair to my hand cycle in my garage and I slowly slid to the ground because my brakes failed. Okay, I thought. I tried for about an hour and a half to get up, with my cell phone right there if I needed to call someone for help. I was able to take the cushion off my chair and use the wall as a brake to hold my chair in place. I was so excited when I did it that I called my cousin Jess to let her know! I do have several people around me with keys to my house in case I fall, so I am very lucky. One morning, I fell getting back into bed at 5 in the morning. I tried to get up for 2 hours and then my arms started shaking, so I called my cousin to come pick me up!

Once I was transferring back to my chair from the toilet, and I ended up on the floor. It wasn't a hard fall; I just slid down the toilet holding the bar on the wall to lessen the impact on my bottom. My roommate left for work, and I said goodbye, not wanting to tell her I was on the floor. She had rescued me a few times after I had fallen, but I was stubborn and wanted to see if I could get off the floor. I worked for about an hour, unsuccessfully, to get back in my chair. My mom and dad happened to be on their way to San Rafael, so they stopped by to pick me up off the ground. Another time, I was taking the garbage out to the curb (my neighbor is so sweet and wheels my yard waste and recycling to the curb each Sunday night). The trash can started wheeling faster than was comfortable, so I attempted to slow it down. When I did that, I dumped myself out of the chair and onto my driveway. Okay. There was no way I would be able to get up on the slant, let alone on a flat surface without a wall to brace my chair. So, I laid there, in my driveway, for approximately two hours, sobbing, intently listening for cars, although surprisingly not cold. Turns out, my neighbor's son in-law stumbled out of the house (a little the worse for wear, I think), so I called to him. Now, my voice is not loud, so I was very thankful he heard me and came next door. I said "I'm paralyzed and fell out of my chair, and I need you to lift me back into my chair." Thankfully, he did it with no problem, and then he moved my trash can to the curb.

I went skiing and had a great time the first round in 2006. I was with two ski instructors at Alpine Meadows near Lake Tahoe who worked well together and must have helped me more as I skied down the slope because I went down the bunny hill at least five times, with seemingly minimal assistance. I was able to ride the chair lift up because I was sitting in a bucket that hinges onto the ski. (One ski: a mono-ski is what I used the first year.) You balance by using the outriggers in each hand, which are ski poles with miniature skis on the ends. When I went again in February 2007 with a group from Santa Clara Valley Med, things didn't go as well.

I had two instructors who did not agree on ways for me to go down the mountain, so I didn't make it onto the chair lift at all. Also, I was put on a bi-ski, not a mono ski like the year before. It had seemed, I'm sure, that I had lost strength, but in reality, my instructors were clashing and thus not helping me. I left the mountain in tears. It is so hard to once be stellar at something and then for it to be such a challenge when you try to do it a different way. I have decided that skiing is not for me: first, because it is too cold; and, two, because it requires the kind of athleticism I just don't have anymore. I always have to remember I am working with one good limb out of four.

As I write, more than five years after the accident, I am seen by the Physical Medicine and Rehabilitation Clinic, Internal Medicine Cline, and the Urology Clinic at UC Davis Med Center. For a pressure sore on my left heel, I've also been treated at Sutter Roseville Hospital, UC Davis Plastic Surgery, and UC Davis Internal Medicine. I continue to do intermittent self-catheterization every four hours, but extending more than seven hours at night. I do a daily bowel program. I do all of my own bathing and dressing. I transfer independently in most situations using a transfer board. I've developed my own physical therapy "programs" by taking courses at the local community colleges. I've seen counselors a number of times, but I realize the true cure for me is to keep busy, just as it always has been my cure.

■   ■   ■

CHAPTER TEN

SPINAL CORD INJURY: LEARNING TO BE A SITTING-DOWN PERSON

"Remember the tea kettle–it is always up to its neck in hot water, yet it still sings."

Anonymous

Every morning when I woke up for that first year, at least those mornings when I was fairly lucid, I forgot where I was and what had happened. I had to remind myself every day that I couldn't just hop out of bed. It was definitely, as "Best Seat in the House" author Allen Rucker put it, "a daily mental adjustment." For those first few months home, in fact, I absolutely refused to believe I was paralyzed. It might have been a way for me to protect myself until I was stronger or it might have been simple, pure denial. In any case, I had to hear the truth from the surgeons who did the original surgery after the accident. Dr. Hunstock, who inserted a steel rod in my back and saw the incredible damage done in April 2004, had to tell me eight months after the accident that I really was paralyzed. He saw me again in January 2005.

I apparently managed to joke about it, though, even early on. My parents and my brother kept track of some of my sillier utterances. At Christmas I peeked in my Christmas stocking and announced, "I don't think there are any legs in here." I always told–and still do tell–the waitresses at restaurants that I have brought my own chair, and I invite my friends and family to pile things on me. "I'm like a cart,"

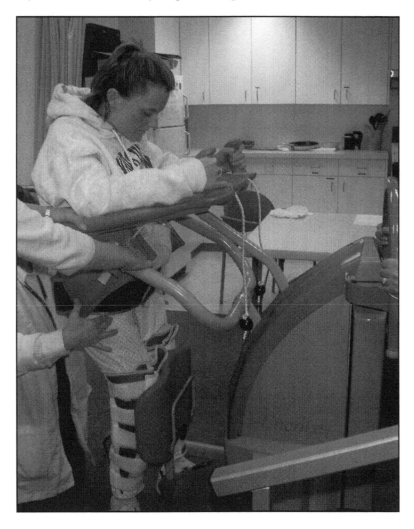

I say. In my first two years, though, I joked and laughed a lot more than I do now.

Sometimes, though, I would say, "I can't wait to get rid of today." And I couldn't.

In a phone conversation with my brother not too long ago, I called myself a "sitting-down person." It makes me laugh and describes me perfectly.

Still, losing the use of my legs is huge and obviously sad. What most people don't know about is the other huge loss that accompanies a spinal cord injury—the ability to manage your bodily functions as easily as everyone else. For me, there's no dashing into a bathroom up a couple steps with narrow entrances and narrower stalls. Sometimes an "accessible" toilet is not accessible. I've been in many bathrooms where I have to pee with the stall door open because my chair doesn't fit with it closed. I've had to pee in the men's urinal because the women's bathroom was upstairs. I've had to pee in a parking lot behind a bush. I've had to pee out the car door several times. I've had to pee into a urinal in bed when camping because it was too complicated to wheel through the site, down the road, all the way to the bathroom. I've had to pee down a hill because there were not-accessible port-o-potties. And, when port-o-potties have been "accessible," the way I pee is facing the toilet and sometimes, the catheter is not long enough to send my pee where it should go: into the toilet. I've had to pee in a portable urinal when the hotel bed was too high to transfer out and pee in the early morning.

Adding insult to injury, I have a condition called

neurogenic bladder. I never feel like I have to pee; I use the clock. Some nurses early on told me I'd get the ability to feel the urge to go again, but they were wrong. Now I set a schedule and have to use a catheter each time I pee. The only advantage over other patients with spinal-cord injury is that I am prescribed the multiple catheters I need as opposed to a few a month like most. Others have to wash and rinse them five times daily for 30 days. Imagine that! And, when the company needs proof that I have this neurogenic bladder, about once a year, I have to make sure my current doctor faxes the form of "medical necessity" to the catheter company. Several times, I've had to rinse my pre-used catheters in bleach water while I'm waiting for the doctor's office to fax the forms the catheter company requires. This is very annoying, especially if I have plans to go anywhere. Thank goodness I've not been blessed with very many urinary tract infections! (The prophylactic antibiotic helps immensely with this.)

The process of catheterization takes a long time. When I first came home, I went through the (initially) hour-long ordeal four times a day: 6 a.m., noon, 6 p.m., and midnight. I would only let my mom help me, so she was back to a schedule similar to one she'd had with us as new babies. She would come at noon every day to catheterize me. She often asked me if I wanted to stay in bed to nap when my eyes looked sleepy. And I often did. I got to take naps every day, but she didn't. My schedule has changed as I've gotten to know my body. I now pee at 5 a.m., 10 a.m., 1 p.m., 5 p.m. and 10 p.m.

If I'm drinking more, I need to pee more. And no caffeine for me. Luckily, I never liked coffee that much.

Eventually I started using the long stretches of time I spent in the bathroom as an opportunity to write in my journal or to talk with friends. For a time, it was a joke that friends only caught me on the phone while I was either in the bathroom or waiting for the bus: Telecare in Grass Valley and Paratransit in Sacramento.

The incredibly specific and not often available physical setting—wider doors, space to roll in front of the toilet, no steps—means that if I want any kind of mobility I have to be ready to pee in some undignified places. I've gone in the back yard at a cousin's in the pouring rain, I've hidden behind a bush and aimed the catheter end down a long hill. I've had to use containers in a car when my parents and I were stuck in traffic. I hate this. A year after the accident, in the summer and into the fall, I kept having lots of peeing accidents, and I really spiraled down. I wrote in my journal that I thought "Alan really got the better end today." It wasn't until I started taking the generic Ditrapan XL (which is supposed to relax my spastic bladder) that my body finally agreed with my pee schedule.

When I visit my brother in San Francisco, I know he is going to have to carry me up the stairs. It's worth it to see him, but I hate being carried up the stairs. He lives on the fourth floor with no elevator, so he'll haul me up and have someone else schlep the chair. Every new trip requires lots of research to see if it is accessible at all.

Taking a shower isn't so easy as it was pre-accident. More than a year after the accident, I started a new journal, and the first entry was a complaint about the weakness in my arm that made for an especially tough transfer into the shower. "It's not fair," I wrote. "My right arm gives me troubles all the time!" We had a chair in the tub at that point. Only recently was the bathroom renovated (again) at my parents' house to accommodate a much easier transfer. But the difficult transfer did make me stronger. They now have a stall shower in a large bathroom with a shower bench. They no longer have a big closet. And, when I am showering there, they always have to make sure to pull the lever which allows the water to flow from the hand-held hose that I use, otherwise, the water would come straight out of the nozzle onto me before it warmed up!

My spinal cord injury has also left me vulnerable to odd infections. About a year and a half after the accident, we discovered a terrible infection in my heel. Of course, I hadn't felt any pain in my foot, although I had stomach cramps so painful they brought tears to my eyes. My foot blew up, though, and my aunt, who is a nurse, saw the red streaks going up the back of my leg. My dad thought it was because I insisted on wearing beautiful, but too tight, shoes.

At the time, I was on Coumadin for a residual blood clot in my leg. The doctor kept increasing the amount of blood thinner so my dosage increased to 10 mg a day from a few milligrams not all the days of the week. Originally, I thought the cramps were because of the high dose of blood thinner. I got a call one night from a doctor at about 11:30 who said my blood was too thin, that I should stop taking Coumadin, and I should try hard not to accidentally cut myself. That call seemed like a crank call at first, but when he started spouting off medical terminology and my personal medical facts, he got my attention.

I ended up in the hospital for a few days because of the infection, but got out in time to fly across country for the first time since the accident. Many weeks later, during a routine appointment, my doctors unwound the wrapping on my foot and told me I'd be spending Christmas in the hospital. "Just cut if off!" I cried. "I don't need it anyway!"

They sent me over to the main University of California Davis hospital emergency room in an ambulance because the rehabilitation doctor thought I would get better treatment. I kept thinking of my last time in an ambulance that I couldn't remember: my mother and I moving from Santa Rosa to Santa Clara Valley Medical Center. Once in the emergency room, I was stuck in a hallway on my bed with a bunch of others hurting in hospital beds. I was finally seen by two doctors, one of whom sliced off about half my heel to spare me gangrene. The sore simply won't go away, though, and I continue to have to treat the sore as a wound.

One really great thing came out of my wrestles with my funky foot. During my emergency room visit in 2006,

I met the great doctor who would become my primary care physician for about two years while she was doing her residency in Sacramento prior to moving back to her home state of Nebraska. She was one of the first (besides the docs at Santa Clara Valley Medical Center) who understood the mix of needs I have because of my traumatic brain injury and spinal cord injury.

I had to buy elastic stockings ($80 for one pair!) With these, I had to be very careful that the bandage stayed on my heel. They're extremely tight stockings, so getting them on was a pain. I slept without them, but I had to put a gauze pad over my sore or else it made extra laundry because my heel sauced all over the pillow with which I elevated my foot. In the shower, I used a wash cloth to clean both feet, spray them with saline, covered the left with a medicated pad, and the right with gauze, then put the stocking on. I am thankful that my problem is with my left foot and not my right because the heterotrophic ossification limits my range leaning to the right. Heterotrophic ossification or HO means there is extra bone growing in my hip where it should not be. Basically, it's your body's way of knowing something has gone terribly wrong; in my case, HO resulted from the head trauma.

Pressure sores are always a problem for paraplegics, although each one is different. Doctors have tried ten or twelve therapies, and my left foot has taken three years to begin to close. But I am now working with a wonderful wound care specialist, Denise, who has closed my left heel wound.

When I brought my cute shoes in to the doctor, for him

and Denise to look at, they instead gave me the cutest pair of moon boots! They are big funky boots with velcro that elevate my heels. I wear them 24-7, except when I am showering.

Denise has been my skin savior since for years. Everyone who has issues like I have had needs a Denise on their team. When she took over for my original doctor handling my wounds, she attacked my sore aggressively, and she took a personal interest in my issues, in ME. It means so much to me that I actually felt bad each time I called her with a new sore. She and I have a connection that really helps me handle all the crap I have to go through because of my injuries.

Denise understands that have the tendency to be quite clumsy, a trait I am really not used to. At my girlfriend's wedding in Clovis in June 2009, I did not have my usual tray I use to carry my tea from the microwave to my table. As a result, I proceeded to spill the almost-boiling water on my thighs just above my knees, which didn't burn, although I could feel it slightly. When my skin started to bubble up, I knew it was bad. My friends Kina and Veronica encouraged me to call Denise. I ended up going to a 24-hour clinic about two minutes from our hotel and then to a nearby pharmacy to get the silvadene cream to dress it each day. I felt so bad for causing yet another wound to my poor body. My body is pretty much falling apart!

In addition to many of the physical challenges of being a sitting-down person, I'm vulnerable to strange remarks and perceptions. People feel free to say things to me that they wouldn't say to someone else, I think. One day as I was waiting for the bus, an older lady glanced at my legs and asked, "Where's your colostomy bag?" I had a hard time believing she was talking to me, but I told her I didn't use one. Another day I was waiting with my legs propped up (my therapists would be proud of me because it was an effort, and I was supposed to do it often), and a much older woman asked me if I were a girl. I had a ball cap on, admittedly, but I did have earrings and lipstick on, too! My roommate Kelly suggested I should have shown her my boobs, but I only had the presence of mind to say a simple yes.

I was wheeling through a mall and a woman was coming down the escalator. She gave me that "poor you" look which is pretty much burned in my brain. In my head I was thinking: 'Poor you, for thinking I am having a crappy life!' Another time when I was at my cousin's graduation from UC Davis law school, the aisle ushers took their jobs a little too seriously, I think. I was parked on the main level just above the bleachers and off the main walkway. I am really not a big person! One of the ushers said I'd need to move to the "designated wheelchair spots." The reason was in the case of a fire, I could not block the aisle. Perfect. My cousin had to fetch my chair at the end of the gym and get me in my chair by lifting me out of the seat.

The worst time, though, was the waitress in the kitchen I had to roll through to reach the accessible bathroom. She shouted: "Make way for the crippled girl!" It took me a second to realize what she said, and then another second to realize she said it about me. (At least she got the gender right.) By the time I was peeing, I just started laughing to myself, painful though it was.

Parties and social situations present some difficulties because there's no way to do any casual mingling in a solid crowd. My chair seems to be a threat–sometimes people stare at my legs and side-step me, with great exaggeration, as if I'm going to run them over! You really hope someone cool decides to come over and chat with you; it's hard having to be more passive. I love being around people, but it is hard to initiate conversation like I used to. I find that different situations are harder for me because of all of the learning that has to happen: especially about where I'm putting stuff. I spend so much time looking for things when I am in new places because their locale is not familiar to me yet.

∎ ∎ ∎

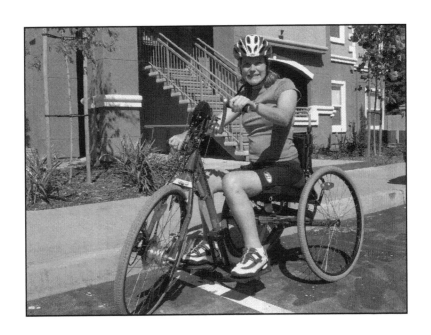

CHAPTER ELEVEN

TRAUMATIC BRAIN INJURY: SHRINKING FEAR

"Expose yourself to your greatest fear, after that, fear has no power, and the fear of freedom shrinks and vanishes. "
Jim Morrison

My paralysis is so visible, but my brain injury has so many more secret problems. If you were to meet me and not know I had a brain injury, you might not guess it. I've shed the glassy eyes and even the uncontrollable giggles I had in the first year or so. At first I didn't talk much, and, when I did, if I wasn't sure about the answer, I would lie and just make something up! What really astonished me because it was something I was not aware of at all was the comment by someone who has known me since 2005. He said to me, in 2009, that I am replying a lot faster to questions or comments from others. That comment really threw me. I thought, 'Was my head injury really that obvious?'

But I continue to have to pressure myself to remember something. As I'm straining, my dad often asks, "Whatcha thinkin'?'" My reply is, "If I wanted you to know, I'd be talkin'!" Typically, though, I am trying to remind myself of the name of the person I'm with, thinking about what I have going on that afternoon, reminding myself of the day and year (yes, this is a scary one), thinking about what I have going on the upcoming weekend (once I figure out what day it is), and trying to remember what I needed to put in my Palm Pilot so I do not forget it.

I've learned how different parts of the brain affect such different things: taste, social screening, memory, organization, bladder, and motor function. Christy listened to a radio show about parts of your brain that control taste, and this is the exact part of my brain that was injured! My taste buds have been altered. I used to love orange juice and wine, and now I cannot stand either! Other things that do not taste good anymore are salmon, yogurt, and bananas. Dan always teases me about my taste buds. It's really pretty funny: I'll say I don't like something and he'll ask teasingly, yet matter-of-factly, 'why?' Another food curiosity is that I like my foods moister than I used to; I prefer to have a dip or sauce on my food. I will never hear the end of it when I decided to dip a piece of American cheese in mustard!

Reading was very hard, and it still is, because I don't have the memory to retain what I've already read. Shorter stories are manageable. Even writing this has been very hard. For the first couple of years, thoughts wouldn't come spontaneously to me, so I had to—and still have to–write in short bursts. My occupational therapist at Sierra Nevada Memorial Hospital, Carin, was the one who first suggested that I think about what I wanted to say as a collection of short stories. I wanted other people with brain damage to be able to read it.

What I hate the most, though, is that I get so panicky when I'm stressed. I don't think clearly when I'm nervous. "I'm always stressed," I said to my brother not long after I got out of the hospital, "but I don't get tired of it." I'd like to be able to manage my money as competently as I used to, but I can't. One time I got a statement on a 401K account I set up when I was working. When I got another statement, I thought I had more money, forgetting completely that I had just gone through the statement. Even now, five years after the accident, I have no idea of what I did and why it was so confusing to me. I'm grateful to be much more able to understand these details—early on in my injury my parents handled everything—but I don't have the comprehension that I used to.

Another brain injury thing that has been frustrating to deal with is that I am not as responsible as I used to be. When I arrived at my aunt's house for dinner on a Sunday night, my cousins came to my car to help me up the curb since I am not good at managing curbs. Well, I decided to leave my purse on the ground leaning against my car. When I came out to the car after dinner, I just thought I had left my purse in the car. I arrived home and looked all around in the car and then in my house. I called my aunt that night and I did a police report. When I checked my bank account, turns out someone had gotten a hold of my purse and had charged 2 things on my account: including a $200 charge, and they cashed a $180 check that I had in my wallet to deposit. I kept thinking: good thing I left my Palm Pilot and pills at home that night! My Palm is my brain! You can imagine what happened to me when I spilled cranberry juice on my Palm. It was like my brain had been put on hold for a while.

This loss presented a slew of things I had to do: replace my ATM and credit cards, driver's license, placard, social security, AAA, insurance, and UC Davis cards. Also, my cell phone was in my stolen purse, so being without a cell for a week was a real pain, especially since I lost all of my numbers. Luckily, my "tech-Dan" brother was able to retrieve all of my stored numbers from the network and reload them onto an old cell phone he gave to me.

My math skills are dreadful, but I honestly probably cannot blame that on my head injury. While I was tutoring sixth graders at my roommate's school once a week, we occasionally worked on math problems. When they'd say the answer, I always would have to quickly calculate in my head, and I struggled mightily. I needed to remind myself, though, that I've never been good with math. To satisfy the college math requirement, I took Math Logic, a course created to help math-challenged people like me graduate.

I'm also not as organized. Things are far more cluttered, although sometimes I launch a fanatical cleaning spree. I know it made my mom crazy as I, newly home again, spread all my things out across my desk and the bar in the kitchen. I can't imagine how I got anything done, but I really wasn't getting much of anything done. My parents were doing all the concentrating for me. Every night they pored over the medical bills and the applications and the health care requirements, exhausted themselves. But I couldn't manage any of it.

My lack of memory and even my doubts about my memory feed my panic. I simply don't trust myself. When I was learning to drive again just before a lesson at my apartment, couldn't find my permit wasn't where it usually is. My driving instructor parked the car and looked everywhere in my apartment for it, with no success. I called my mom, afraid she had cleaned it out. I finally found it in a different purse.

Forgetting things continues to be the common theme in my life, although my memory does continue to improve.

My friend Kelly handed me the tickets to a River Cats game in Sacramento. We got up to the gate, and I insisted I didn't have them, so she had to run back to the car—probably almost a mile away. Meanwhile I was supposed to be waiting in line. By the time she got back, I realized I had the tickets. I'm lucky my friend is a patient soul, but I apologized profusely anyway. I hate not remembering.

When I first got home to Grass Valley, I was looking at something new with my parents, mystified by my ownership. "I know I didn't steal them, I just don't remember buying them," I said.

Another curious side effect of traumatic brain injury is that I fixate on minute details that I used to not care about. My senses for symmetry and order are super-powered now: if a picture is crooked on the wall, if your tie is off center, I will notice and mention something about it.

Mentioning things I wouldn't have mentioned is a problem, too. I used to pride myself on being polite. Now I blurt things out: "You're a baby," I said to a 23-year-old at my apartment complex. And, my friend Sarah got married in early June and her new last name is Peelo. Well, I misheard her over the phone, thinking she said her new last name would be "Kilo." I blurted out: my first dog's name was Kilo. How cool is that to be compared to a freakin' dog? It's not so bad saying things so haphazardly, it's just embarrassing.

I get the hiccups often. They are quite annoying. And, whenever I drink, I cough. For some reason, I cannot swallow a liquid without coughing. Believe me, I have tried.

I also yawn all the time. I do not know if this is my brain injury, but I do know that it is awful. I know that one of my lungs was bruised by Harvey and I wonder if that is part of the reason why I cannot get enough oxygen to my lungs.

My singing voice, which once was beautiful and clear, seemed to take a hit, although I don't know if it's to do with my brain or my spine. My widowed aunt recently remarried, and I sang with other people for the first time in public. I was told I sounded fine, but I've got no "head voice" anymore.

I get sad when I'm overtired, and I get overtired more easily given my brain injury. My mood goes way down and I hate it; it's like I'm very deep in a well and cannot escape. I'm drowning with no way out. My typical reaction is that I feel hopeless. My swinging emotions affect those around me too. Often, when I'm in this sort of funk, I curse Harvey. If only he could hear what I say to him!

When I was still in the hospital in Santa Clara, I started to cry myself when a group of TBI and SCI patients returned from dinner at Bucca di Beppo in Campbell. "What's wrong, Jill? Didn't you have fun going to dinner with us?" Dan asked me. I told him I was upset because "I had to ride in the crazy van. I know I'm a little bit crazy at times, but the other patients are all nuts." I was one of the crazy ones, of course.

For a long time, I couldn't control my laughter. Some traumatic brain injury patients have anger problems. I felt lucky to have laughter problems, but it was still a problem. I couldn't help myself giggling uncontrollably in the middle of conversations, couldn't follow the conversation well enough for anything to match up. The laughter covered a lot. But as my brain heals, this laughter is replaced with more serious feelings: feelings about what Harvey took from me. I miss Alan so much.

Many SCI patients also have trouble with regulating body temperatures. Many are hot all the time, which would be very annoying because it's harder to cool off than get warm–everyone has to wear clothes! I am always cold. It never fails. One weekend, Dan and I were riding in the car with our Aunt Paula and Uncle Bill when our parents were in Calistoga with their friends on an annual trip. Driving back from having dinner in San Francisco in the early winter, I was cold, as usual. With great chivalry, Bill said he wouldn't turn off the heater until I was warm. We got to their house in San Rafael after being in the 109-degree car for about 15 minutes. It felt great to me, but everyone else was sweating.

The chill I feel constantly is not like a typical chill others feel. The chill is to the bone; I always have a shudder in my body. Curiously, even though I am cold always, my legs feel hot to the touch. On my bed, I have a feather mattress cover, sheets, feather comforter, and down throw blanket. I always sleep with a sweatshirt on. Although it took three years for me to realize, if I wear socks to bed, I'm warmer. Sometimes I even sleep with a beanie on my head. When I go to my parents' house in Grass Valley, my mom has piled six blankets on the bed because she knows I get cold. It still feels weird to have that many blankets on my bed.

In spite of that, my butt gets hot. It gets tired of sitting all the time. I am half tempted to get in bed and lie on my side to reduce the pressure on it. I remember when I was not doing weight shifts very often (or very well), and it would never get sore. Maybe it's because I am more aware of the importance of weight shifts and how they help prevent sores: I got a sore on my butt that caused my wound care specialist to send me to the hospital. For 3.5 days I was in the hospital, with no shower, laying on a special air bed they ordered for me. I had ultrasounds, MRIs, and x-rays to make sure my sore was not to the bone. It wasn't.

Things that help:

Initially, I think it helped my brain to force my arms and hands to move. My dad gave me a ball long before I had a clue what a ball was and made me squeeze it.

Once I came back to the world of the conscious, people gave me "tasks" to accomplish with my memory. My brother made me remember his engineering class titles, my friend Danh made me remember to call him weekly (which I still do). My speech therapist in Grass Valley had me remember a newspaper story each day and a quote for a week. On a vacation in April 2007, Dan gave me another challenge: to think about moving my legs every day. Yeah. We'll see if that one happens.

The quotes I remembered from my speech therapy in Grass Valley from January 2005 to August 2006, a year to two years after the accident, that follow directly were from the book *Safe Passage*. I remembered them visually. As an example, the first quote I had to remember, I pictured my wrist for a watch, my legs for feeling (since I have none), and my heart for "loved one." It is interesting the games you play to remember something.

Men, coffee, chocolate. The stronger the better. (I changed rich to strong.)

The something that is not lost, even when the other person is gone, is the self. This may be an ending, but it is not the end.

I can look into the world and see you in every act of love. Where once you were one, you are now many.

I started missing you long before you were gone. I'll keep loving you long after the memories bring you back.

You are not lost. You continue in every hearty laugh, in every nice surprise, and in every reassuring moment in my life.

Death has separated us but not completely. We have not parted company forever. I'm only living away from you for a while.

Everything precious including our dignity can be taken from us but the one thing that can't be taken away is our power to choose what attitude we will take toward the events that have happened.

What is immutable is love and its sheer power. Not even death can diminish its possibilities.

Thank you for being part of my life. It's time to move on. I bow inwardly to the memory of you and, turning away, face the new day.

I can do something marvelous with my grief. Despite everything that has happened, despite even death, I can still love you and will still love others.

Alongside the one goodbye we recognize so well, so many others can be heard, a chorus of parting that is happening all over the world.

Life will not go on in the same way without him. The fact that he left behind a place that cannot be filled is a high tribute to the uniqueness of his soul.

Play for more than you can afford to lose, and you will win the game.

It's not the number of breaths you take, but the times that take your breath away. (My favorite: I used this quote on my website a few times by accident.)

. . .

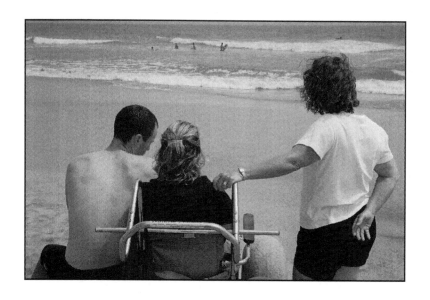

CHAPTER TWELVE
GRIEF

"All the flowers of all the tomorrows are in the seeds of today."
Anonymous

Sometimes people ask me for what I grieve the most, and the answer is always Alan. But he's at the top of a long list I try not to take out of the mental drawer too often. I miss my legs, I miss my memory, I miss running, I miss swimming, I miss my quickness, I miss my time. I hate being cold. I hate being stared at. I hate giggling uncontrollably. I miss my backless shoes and my short shorts and dresses. When I was going to donate all of my shoes that were stored in a big box in my garage, I looked at them and got tears in my eyes. One man had caused me to have to give up all of these shoes that I have had wonderful times in!

Some people ask if there's anything they can do, and when I've got the list in front of me, I think, yes, sure, you can turn back time, take away my pain, and bring Alan back. Not possible? Then just be on my side while I face the demons. And I'm fortunate to have so many people on my side to help me. I recently went to a group for people coping with grief, and it helped me. One meeting, I actually broke down and cried, which was one of a handful of times I have been able to cry about the losses. I think telling the new group of my story was a wake-up call to my body saying: 'Hey! You've lived through this, and why aren't you sad outwardly about it?' But as time goes on, I am much more able to control these emotions, and when I am feeling sad about things, I can cry, which feels so good. But I do cry over the smallest things, yet another blessing of the brain injury!

A couple of years after we were hit, my dad's cousin Sally wrote and asked me a question I'm still trying to answer. She believes that nothing happens "by accident," although "that reason may be obscured, sometimes for years. Events that seem horrible at the onset turn out to be necessary lessons that are blessings in disguise. One not only learns to accept them, but eventually to embrace and be grateful for them because the growth and wisdom they provoke wouldn't or couldn't have occurred otherwise. In the years since your life was shattered and derailed so horribly, and so unfairly, have you found this to be at all true? I hope so." I hope so, too. I don't know yet. Sometimes, before I got to sleep at night, I lay there and think that maybe Alan is watching me from above, talking to me and telling me to move on, things are getting better, and "I am watching you, so make me proud!" I picture the bedroom door opening and having his brilliant smile peeking into me.

One would guess that I would be a complete mess. And, sometimes, I feel like that: totally ready to stay in bed all day and put the covers over my face. I was not physically able to cry for at least a year after the accident. (I would giggle instead.) My flood gates opened–and it felt good–and haven't stopped. The problem with these flood gates is that I have a hard time regulating them. For example, when I am especially stressed about something or overtired, I tend to cry more, feel like my life is hopeless, and say that Alan got the better end of the deal (which nobody wants to hear).

I have had to realize that my emotions do whatever they want. I constantly find myself cursing Harvey, sometimes out loud. Once, when it was raining and I was going over to the computer center at night (before I had email at home), I imagined myself wheeling straight into the pool. Rash and way overreacting; I chalked it up to my head injury.

In addition to times when I am stressed, I am more easily upset if I don't have a lot on my plate and am bored. This isn't a new development in my life, however. I've never dealt well with boredom. When these moods hit me, talking to my family really helps—although I also feel like they have to take the brunt of my negativity. I've realized that if I do not have a solid plan for a day, I feel like my life is worthless. What the hell am I doing here? That's what I feel. One of my old therapists used to always talk about "doing things in the community." I thought the idea was lame, but I'm beginning to realize that integrating myself helps me to shift focus off the bad parts of my life.

My favorite counselor, Emily, helped me understand how I was wasting a lot of energy beating up myself. One of my first thoughts when I realized I had just "wasted" five months in the hospital was how upset my mother must have been by my being so unproductive. Crazy! Our family has always set a store on working hard, and here I was not contributing! Emily had me make a list of my self-made critiques:

> You used to be so fast, now it takes you forever just to get dressed.
>
> You used to be as sharp as a tack.
>
> Your life was so perfect! I think it was going too well.
>
> What's your right hand doing?
>
> Sit up straight, and don't have that blank stare!
>
> Why can't you remember this?
>
> Why don't you understand what people's mouths are saying?
>
> People are looking at me in a chair and wondering 'What's wrong with her?'
>
> Then we worked together to figure out ways to combat these critiques:

Talk back to your hopeless critic:

Your brain keeps healing

You will get faster

You will find someone as wonderful as Alan–hold out for open, athletic, smart, charismatic, confident, happy, honest, loyal

Things aren't as bad as you think they are

You have a wonderful family and group of friends

When you feel insulted, take some time to remember 17 other times someone has complimented you.

Don't worry about wasting your time; wasting time is brain time because it gives your brain time to rest and wonder.

Know that sadness–and boredom–are part of your recovery.

Remember you have grey zones, in-between steps when approaching new situations

Develop an action plan and write it down: Find a living situation, figure out your insurance, plan to re-learn driving and get a car, and dream about your next job.

Keep a journal by your bed to record dreams.

Wake up thinking you may be slower than before the accident, but you're faster than you were six months ago. You're strong and active and you have goals to accomplish.

Listen to music to get your energy going.

Think of one thing you are looking forward to.

Remember it's fine to tell people you don't need help.

Remember that April 11 is also the day you survived; you surprised everyone who thought it was hopeless; it was the beginning of your new life.

Some advice wasn't as helpful to me. One caregiver I had in Sacramento insisted that if I "fully believed in God, He can heal." Although I didn't say anything to her, I thought to myself that my faith must be sadly lacking or I wouldn't be in such a fix. (This makes me laugh again each time I read it, remembering how sure she was of this advice!)

I'm sometimes sad about how I spend my time. For the first three years after the accident, all time was spent recovering or waiting to recover. When I gained some independence and moved to Sacramento, I basically divided my time among waiting for the special bus, peeing, and sitting on the phone with insurers defending my need for counseling, and catheters. Sometimes I still don't understand how even though I'm not working, I'm so busy I hardly have time to work on this book! Everything takes so long.

One of the few good things early on was that I was never bored. It took nearly three and a half years for me to regain any sense of being bored–and then, like a child, I would pick fights with my parents.

Early on I was not particularly sad, either. My mom, the counselor and intuitive woman she is, says that this is the way my body protects me from my losses: Alan, the use of my legs, my job, my brain, and my old life. I even refused to believe I was paralyzed. I woke up every morning and had to remember again. I made a little deal with myself: I would believe my paralysis true and enduring only after I heard it from the two doctors, Alan Hunstock and Eldan Eichbaum, who had laid eyes on my damaged spinal cord and completed the surgery. I guess it was a way for me to put off the bad news until I could handle it and start anew: once they told me I would never walk again, I would know it was fact. Dr. Hunstock gave me the bad news, again, eight months after the accident in January 2005. I talked to him again in 2007, and he said my case was the worst he had seen in all his years of practice.

Some days I am still incredibly angry at Harvey for what he did. I probably won't ever understand how someone can be so drunk that he could smash two bicyclists before noon on an Easter Sunday. Many people have asked if I ever want to meet him. I decline: saying he is not worth my time, and because of him, my time is quite valuable. About a year after the accident, though, I wrote him a letter. Writing helped. Still, I didn't actually send the letter.

April 2005
Harvey Hereford
Department of Corrections
San Quentin Prison

I saw you for the first time in the Santa Rosa court, and I was scared to see you. Scared that I would lose my temper and jump out of my chair to attack you, if I could. But your carelessness has left me bound to a wheelchair most likely for the rest of my life. You also took away my best friend. His family and I will never forgive you. Alan's grandmother was so right in court when she said that "you do not deserve to breathe the same air we breathe." I hope you never forget what she said to you. But most likely, you will forget because that's just who you are.

I tried to tell you in court what I miss and the things that used to be so easy for me that now are major obstacles. But I am sure you weren't listening very closely. It's hard for me to talk to my friends and adults who can still walk. They always have to look down on me. This is something I never thought of about people in wheelchairs. I have friends and family who I can tell this—and luckily they understand because they are my friends and family. I constantly say "What do people do who don't have the support system I've had through this ordeal?" I have been very lucky.

What was published in the Santa Rosa Press Democrat was not what I wanted to say. You can't even put into words how furious I am. And having a master's degree in Mass Communications helps me to be very educated about language. Some days are just so hard for me, and I used to be such a happy-go-lucky person all the time.

Another thing I really miss, besides Alan, is my independence. Because I am not strong enough yet, I have to be in my chair all the time if no one is home. This means that I need to be out of bed if anyone is to leave me alone. And I have only stayed alone for a handful of times. When my parents leave, they always call someone to say that I'll be here alone. This is really hard because I was so used to being independent when I wasn't with my friends or with Alan.

You also hurt my parents and brother; if not physically, then emotionally. I am now an around-the-clock burden for them. And I hate it. To give you an example, we went camping for the Fourth of July and we had to drive up to Redding—Lake Shasta—to see if the site was accessible for me. Whenever anyone plans a trip—and we have a lot—we need to make sure that the place is accessible for me. I am very lucky that I have huge support through all of this. I am lucky to have the friends and family I have.

I find myself wondering what I did to deserve this punishment. And what did Alan do that was so bad? But then I realize that it is not because Alan or I did something wrong; it's because you weren't conscious enough to think before you got behind the wheel that morning on April 11, 2004.

Now, time rules my life and it was your action that made it become the dominant force. I always have to be aware of the time to empty my bladder. The way I do it is with a catheter. Luckily, I've started doing it into the toilet but I used to have to empty my bladder in bed every four hours. And speaking of that, I've had many accidents which are annoying to everyone involved. This problem makes me feel like a kid again. This sucks!

I do have a few happy moments. Like when I walk in the parallel bars with braces strapped on my legs. To give you an idea, I've had to relearn how to move my body around. Because my legs were always the strongest part of my body, I've had to pay close attention to my arms. Unfortunately, my arms have never been as strong as my legs, even though I was an athlete. Another added frustration is the brain injury caused my right—dominant—hand and arm to be numb so it makes things extra hard when I want to use it which is often because my legs don't work anymore. In the hospital, the therapists said, "When you can give the finger to anyone that will be great."

I also think about my relationship with Alan. A lot of my friends and family said that he seemed to be the one. I thought so too because we had so much in common. I think about our time together and I think there will never be another man like him. So that's another thing you can think about in jail: the life I will lead without him and the life of his that you took away.

Before this injury, I had enough money saved up to buy a house. Thank goodness I didn't because there would be no way for me to pay for it now. I loved my job. Loved my boyfriend. And loved my life. In court I was so right when I said that you took my life away even if your stupidity didn't kill me. I hope you have lots of time to think about the injury you caused and how you truly affected us and our families.

Jill C. Mason, M.S.

■　■　■

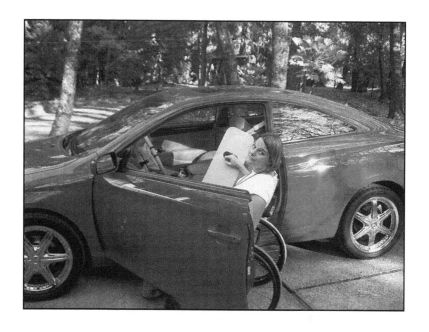

CHAPTER THIRTEEN

MOBILITY:
TRAVELING TO THE FUTURE

"You'll learn more about the road by traveling it than consulting all the maps in the world."

Anonymous

I loved to run, I loved to swim, and I loved to cycle. I loved the power of my own body and the freedom. But now I've got to power external machines to get myself my freedom.

And my independence. Without mobility, I never would have made it to independence.

Here's the inventory of what I use and what I've tried to keep me mobile:

Car

Standing frame: Helps promote circulation by standing me up

Wheelchair with red spokes to match my car

Hand cycle

CHAIRS

As I was preparing to leave the hospital, my therapists put me in an electric wheelchair so I could learn to use it. The hand controls were on the left side because my left hand was stronger and more capable. My brother wasn't happy about the electric aspect of the wheelchair or the fact that my right hand would sit unused while the left got stronger. He and my friend Danh spent one evening at Santa Clara Valley Medical Center shifting the controls to the right side after they figured out the wiring. Two engineers–they managed fine. Then they took me out to the patio and ordered me around like a couple of drill sergeants. Not that their orders mattered–my right hand was, as expected, not very effective in controlling the wheelchair, and I careened around in the darkness, laughing. I ended up doing a death spiral in a fit of laughter. But after all of this, I learned faster.

Insurance bought me an electric wheelchair. I used it on walks down my parents' road and once to go to the Rite

Aid by my apartment in Sacramento. Here's the thing about the electric wheelchair, though: it makes me feel paralyzed and I don't like it. When I use it, I feel lazy. Yes, it's great for getting places fast, but I have a prejudice against it. It's got some practical considerations against it, too: it won't fit into my car, my friends' cars, and it won't go over steps. And, what happens if it runs out of juice when you are out? There is no way to manually push it.

My insurance also provided money for a manual wheelchair. Insurance, however, would not authorize a titanium chair, and I couldn't haul the heavier chair into my car. I ended up spending about $5,000 to to buy my red-spoked titanium chair.

The transition at home wasn't easy. I started out slowly. The first wheelchair I was prescribed after getting out of the hospital was a disaster. We had to wait for it to arrive, and then the size was all wrong. It was uncomfortable and heavy. It took me at least ten minutes to push from the kitchen to my bedroom at my parents' house, a distance of about 40 feet.

With the wheelchair not right, my first sessions learning to transfer from the bed to the chair were hard. They would have been hard even with a good right hand and arm!

I discovered that the most important thing for any new wheelchair user is fit and weight. While I keep my old wheelchair as a backup, what I use is my titanium chair. The titanium keeps it light enough for me to swing the body of the chair across me and into the car's passenger seat. When I drive, I have to flip the chair on its side, pull off the wheels by pushing the middle, and put the wheels and cushion on the passenger seat floor. I use the bar on the ceiling of my car to lift the body of the chair over me sitting on the reclined passenger seat. This took about ten minutes for a few years (less than five minutes five years later!) but it still is awful in the rain!

Tires are more of a problem because they go flat, and it's usually when I'm in a hurry to get somewhere I want to go. Not long ago, my mom and dad and I were headed to San Jose to visit my friend Sarah for her birthday, but the red chair's tire was flat. I was angry because I had to wheel around in my old chair with the high back and skinny hand grips on the wheels. My old chair makes me feel like I am unruly and totally backwards. I overreacted, cursing Harvey and wishing he would have just taken me, too. My parents endured all this, as they have so much else. We didn't go to Sarah's party, but we ended up meeting my brother and his fiancee in San Francisco, and I calmed down. I now keep two extra wheels in my house with the tire pumped and two extra tubes in my trunk.

As I was getting my chair out of the car and putting it together for class one day, I put the wheel down on something sharp. It started leaking air fast, but I managed to get home after my workout and exchange the wheel. My brother came the next day to visit, and he fixed the tires for me. I don't know what I'd do without my family!

I think at times I may have gotten somewhat used to

being in the chair, but I had a bad moment one day as I watched my dad coming out of the driveway sitting in my electric chair. We were in Grass Valley before I moved to Sacramento, and I was doing laps in my hand cycle at the top of the road, working on my arm strength. As I was working out, I glanced down the road to see him coming toward me, and it scared me because for a moment I imagined he needed the chair to move. Poor Mom and Dan, I thought in a flash. But Dad was just making sure the chair was still charged. Still, the moment gave me a bad turn, nonetheless.

STANDING FRAME

I've been fortunate enough to have a standing frame. It's expensive, and, like the titanium, was not covered by insurance, so my grandmother bought it for me. It essentially stands me up and increases my circulation. I get so tired of sitting on my butt all the time. The first time I tried one was at Santa Clara Valley Medical Center during my rehabilitation, and my first comment was: "I'm so tall!" All 5'2" of me!

BIKES

My bike is a three-wheeled hand cycle, and I absolutely hate it when people call it a trike. I know that's technically what it is, but give me a break! The pedals are level with my chest. To brake, I pull back on the pedals—so no reverse. It's the same height as my chair so I transfer into it without a board and always wear my helmet. My friends Erin and Jeff gave me a motorcycling flag to affix onto the back of my bike so I am more visible to cars. I usually ride around my neighborhood for a little over an hour. I love the freedom it provides. Also, there is a bike path I like just a half mile from my place. Typically, I go with my brother or parents, and they speed walk or jog while I push. Going uphill is very hard because you're essentially pulling up your whole body and the bike with your arms alone. I've only accomplished that once, with Dan's encouragement.

I went once to Yosemite with a Sacramento sporting group, Access Leisure. The week was filled with riding and camping. Now, I really was not slow prior to my injury, but I was by far the slowest of the sporting group. The group had really great riders who would go on 20-mile bike rides twice a day. I so wanted to be as fast and with their endurance. Unfortunately, I could not hang. The furthest I went was 7.5 miles one day to Fallen Leaf Lake, and my friend rode behind me up the incline to give me a great deal of help up the last mile or so. At the top, it was beautiful, but I got into the van there, because there was no way I had the energy to cycle all the way back to camp.

I also went to a cycling event that was held at Discovery Park. I ended up riding about 8 miles on one of the bike paths. I rode back with one of the employees because, as usual, I was not as fast as the group–and I was in the slower group. Turns out, the bike seat was not right for my skin, so I developed a pressure sore on my right butt cheek that I had to treat by laying down every day for about a month. Maybe one had been starting, maybe not, but either way, I was checking my butt one time and I found it. I was pretty much falling apart! My knees were burnt, my heals had sores, and my butt was going to fall off! So, no summer school for me! This is when I came the closest to losing it all together.

I worked on my book while sitting on the toilet because I could sit up without sitting on anything. When my parents and brother came down for father's day, I was a real brat and I attribute that to having no endorphins going since I was lying down all the time. So, on a roll we took when they were here, I decided that rolling, not riding on my bike, for about an hour a day would do my attitude good and not hurt my butt too much. Plus, getting my blood pumping I'm sure would help heal all my war wounds.

CARS

It's my car, though, that's bought me hours of freedom. No more waiting for other people or the bus. No more rolling a mile or two on Sacramento sidewalks getting from one appointment to another. First, though, I had to learn to drive and then to prove to the State of California I was capable of driving. Two years after the accident, I hired a service called Bond Driving School in Sacramento to help me learn how to drive a car only with my hands.

The hand controls are on the left of the steering wheel: down controls the gas and forward controls the brake–dangerous if you forget which does which thing! This tool is a lever like a turn signal. The controls can be mounted on any automatic car in a matter of a few hours. It's quite ingenious, and anyone qualified can drive with these controls.

I tried two methods of steering, the knob and the V-shaped tool on the steering wheel. The knob is better for me because I don't have to adjust my hand too much for the turns. Basically, I just need to use my upper body strength and have souped-up power steering. Power steering is vital in any car because you need the strength to turn at the same time you are accelerating or braking. I learned on a car with limited power steering and really struggled. During my driver's test with DMV, I was with a tester who was new. She told me where to go on the back streets by DMV, and then I asked her when we were getting on the freeway? Slightly shocked, she asked, "Do you want the right to travel on the freeway?" Hmmm. It was a good thing I asked because it is impossible to get to see most of my friends and family without going on the freeway! If I hadn't have tested on the freeway, I would have had yet one more restriction on my license: "No freeway."

When I first announced my goal of driving and getting a vehicle, everyone kept asking me if I were going to get a van. NO!! I knew that right away. I simply didn't want to look like a handicapped-van person. It turned out that there were plenty of choices. My parents patiently took me to countless car dealers so I could see how easily I could transfer. I originally wanted a Mazda RX8 with a "suicide door" that allows for a very wide opening so I can more easily get my chair into the back seat. However, the Mazda was just too low for me to transfer easily.

I was very happy with my final choice, a Toyota Solara. I roll to the door, transfer in, put the cushion on the floor of the passenger seat between the wheels. Then I lean my seat back and flip the chair body onto the passenger seat, resting the big bar against the glove box.

Not long after I got my new car, I smashed my new car. I was pulling out of a parking lot and thought I'd make it across the intersection as the light turned yellow, the typical California stop. Then I realized—too late–that the car ahead of me was stopping because he wouldn't have made it across the road; there were too many cars. In my head I blamed my slow reaction time on my head injury, but I've been reminded that other people have exactly the same stupid accidents, and they don't have a head injury to blame. So I did it, and I was crushed. In shock, I pulled into a Ford dealership, and they helped me with everything. About two weeks later, and after paying a hefty insurance deductible, my car came back to me.

In the meantime, I rented another hand-controlled car. Nothing's easy with any accident. Many, many lost hours on the phone and the additional challenge of finding a car with hand controls. I was beside myself, so my parents came down from Grass Valley to Sacramento that night. Once we got the rental car, they made me drive on the freeway. I got back in the saddle, but the collision did make me far less cocky. I remind myself that I'm not as quick as I used to be. I drive like an old lady now, letting down the image of the young chick in the red sports car!

TRAVELING

I'm getting faster and faster in my daily life. I can get in and out of the car, do my errands, visit my friends, get myself to my speaking engagements and doctor's appointments.

Traveling is manageable, but a little more problematic. I've learned a few things each time I get on the plane and stay in strange places.

Basically, when I fly, I watch my liquid intake! Airplane bathrooms are impossible to enter with a wheelchair. Besides, to get into the plane, you would need the aisle chair (which is tiny) and have to pee with the door open because they are so small. I took a five-hour flight to Hawaii to visit my girlfriend Kina and managed just fine, but I was pretty thirsty.

Seat assignment is hugely important. After my family boarded our first cross-country flight, we realized we didn't have any aisle seats, something absolutely necessary for a wheelchair user. I also needed the arm rest raised so I could transfer into the seat. And, unfortunately, the button that allows you to do that is obscure, even to most airline attendants! The flight attendants asked an aisle-seated lady to switch with me, but she refused to move, loudly proclaiming how hard she had fought for the seat. Hearing this, I started to cry. Everything finally worked out, but we had a few cheerless moments. I also usually need assistance getting into the seat.

Hotels and motels, even those billing themselves as handicapped-accessible, are not always prepared. Several places I've stayed have scrambled to provide a bath bench for me to use in the shower. They've had to go buy them on the spot. Once I rolled into a beautiful shower at a motel only to flood the entire bathroom because the water rolled out of the shower. So my family had to brush their teeth that night while standing in a puddle. My mother left a pretty harsh critique.

Bed heights are another challenge. Hotels think higher beds are fancier, but I can't get in or out of them without lots of help. I headed to my girlfriend's wedding in Clovis and drove down there with my other girlfriend who is very strong and sweet, but I hoped so much that the bed height would not be an issue so I could be as independent as possible. Turns out, it was pretty high, and each time I transferred in or out, someone was spotting me! So, when I peed at five a.m., I just went into a urinal so I did not have to wake anyone up to help me transfer. Ah, the joys of being paralyzed!

Even getting into bathrooms can be a problem. Sometimes I can get in, but I've had to roll through the kitchen in a restaurant or the back alley or some other nasty place just to get where I'm going at all. Oh, you need the "accessible" bathroom? Just roll through all of this trash and then you will find the accessible bathroom! Then when you get in, the toilet is in the wrong place. We stayed in a beach house for a few days where I had to pee sideways and do the bowel program in the bedroom. At a Giants' game in San Francisco in May 2009, I went to the bathroom before we went into the stadium while we were tailgating. They had an accessible port-o-potty, however, "accessible" seemed to be a loose term. The way I pee is facing the toilet with my legs on each side of the bowl. However, there was no way for me to get my legs through the hard plastic of the port-o-potty, so thank goodness my catheter was long! (Sorry if that was TMI!) Anyway, while I was dealing, the lock on the door did not work properly so someone busted the door open. They did not apologize to ME, they simply said "There's a wheelchair in there." Hmmm. There was a PERSON in there as well! Ugh.

As a family, we've basically learned that we are more comfortable, on the whole, staying in hotels when we visit friends and family. This is something we never would have done before the accident. I feel horrible that this is the case, but if I'm not happy, I have a tendency to be almost impossible to be around. When I need more help, I do not like it. Because of my head injury, I'm much more comfortable at home and in a familiar setting. I know this frustrates people because they work so hard to make things work for me.

. . .

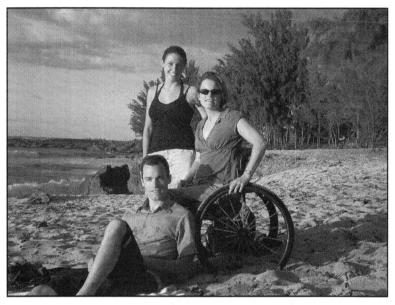

Jill, her brother Dan, and his fiancee, Melanie, in Oahu, Hawaii, in 2007.

CHAPTER FOURTEEN

INDEPENDENCE: GROWING UP AGAIN

"Slight not what's near, while aiming at what's far."
Euripides, 'Rhesus'

When I was first hurt, the initial prognosis was gloomy, and the word "independent" was not in anyone's vocabulary. Death or a kind of twilight life was the initial expectation for me. Even after I moved home, expectations were not high that I would ever attain any independence approaching that I had known before. For me, independence combines living away from my parents and working at something productive. It's taken years, but I'm living in Sacramento, speaking and volunteering at various places and trying to sort out what job I'd like to do in the future.

Before the accident, I was actively looking to buy a condominium or house near the job I loved. I looked at one place with a yard and at another in a building with stairs that now would be completely unmanageable. Alan and I went to a few open houses together. Since the accident, I've lived in the hospital, at home with my parents, in an apartment with a roommate, and, finally, in my own house.

Before I found my apartment, my parents helped me look for a long time. We saw practically every new and old apartment complex in the nice areas of Sacramento. The apartment we found was perfect—I had my own huge bathroom I could maneuver around in my chair, a porch I could roll to, and plenty to see from our porch. The kitchen in our apartment was great with the oven and stove controls on the front, the microwave on the counter, a cut-out sink, and lowered pantry shelves. Kelly, my roommate in the apartment for two years, was a mutual friend of one of my lacrosse friends. She is a kindergarten teacher, and a very dedicated one at that, always bringing work home to prepare for activities for her class.

The complex was so new that, in fact, Kelly and I

rented one of the first apartments. Initially, the apartment manager moved us into a temporary apartment because ours was not completed. This ended up being a good thing because I was able to do a walk-through (well, a roll-through) with the construction guys and tell them exactly what worked for me in the apartment. So, the accessibility was ideal for me. The pool even had a mechanized lift that I used occasionally. It was, however, a pain in the butt to be all wet and cold from the pool and then roll back to my apartment to shower and change. Things in a chair are never as easy. A shopping center was within an easy rollable distance. In fact, I worked with the shopping center property manager to install a cement pathway directly from my apartment complex to the neighboring shopping center, which was very convenient once it was installed. We discovered that many places billed as handicapped-accessible really weren't. My parents and I needed to visit each one.

In 2008, I decided I wanted my own place and started looking in February, sometimes with my realtor friend and sometimes with my parents. After looking for about six months, I finally found my home on my birthday, July 9, 2008, in the South area of Sacramento. I immediately called my parents to come down and take a look: this was the one. It is in a great neighborhood just next to the Sacramento River. I have the best neighbors who so sweetly help me manage my trash, yard waste, and recycling cans each week. My realtor's husband is a contractor, so he was able to do all of the modifications that I needed to have done: bars, cut out sinks, and removal of a few doors. I also hired someone to create ramps for me that do not make it look like a handicapped person lives in the house.

To help with the mortgage, I have a roommate, a police officer who works three twelve-hour shifts out of the South Sacramento office. He lives in the front of the house. He tells me sometimes about all of the impaired drivers he pulls over.

I've now started to ponder my working future. Humans need to work and feel productive, in addition to the social aspects of work. I used to be a marketing professional. I'm not anymore, but I didn't discover that right away. I attended a career fair in Sacramento in the late summer of 2008 and realized that each job I was interested in required a different degree that my master's in mass communications. It was more than annoying to be made to feel like my degree means nothing because my life has been changed so drastically.

That year I was released from the hospital, 2004, I took my brother as a date to my old company holiday party. It was my first major public outing, I think, and we closed the party down. We were so loud when we came back to the hotel room that we woke my parents, who had brought me down because I needed so much help. My voice had been very soft up to that point, but my mom pointed out that I seemed to have found some volume that night.

I did the company slideshow the next year for the holiday party with Erin, but by the following year, two years after I'd left the company, I didn't know enough people to be of much help. I understood then that I would not be going back. The time had come to move on emotionally.

More important, though, I had to face what I could do and what I wanted to do.

Nearly two years after the accident, I wrote a simple invitation and proofed it properly. My cousin Jess had me design and print her wedding shower and bachelorette party invitations. The project felt good to accomplish. And little did she know that her trust in my work was very important to me. My work skills disappeared in the instant I was hit, but some have been coming back in fits and starts. My brother's fiancée, Melanie, is having me do her bridal shower and bachelorette invitations for December 2009. I really like this work: using photos and colors to make an invitation visually appealing. I guess that is a part of my marketing background that has stayed with me.

About a year after the accident I decided I wanted to start speaking with school children about drunk drivers. Something good needed to come of what had happened, and I wanted to keep teenagers from driving drunk. I painstakingly put together a slideshow. Sometimes I was furious with my progress and my brain injury. Something I could have finished in an hour was taking days. As I updated slides, I would forget what I'd already done. My brother Dan helped me initially clean up the slides, adding in some more pictures of me and Alan before and of me alone after the accident. I am very involved in the Every 15 Minute programs that most high schools have for juniors and seniors. Schools select about 30 students to wear black with white painted faces and be totally apart from any school interaction, as if they have been killed by a drunk driver. They are taken out of class and removed from every aspect of school and their family and friends for about 24 hours. They go away on a retreat, (at which I present as well) when they are taken away from their homes for a night as if they are really dead: killed by a drunk driver. At the assembly the following day, typically a casket is paraded through the gym behind a bagpiper to the front near all of the "dead" students who are sitting in chairs facing the audience. At many of these assemblies, the whole school is absolutely silent, and this is when I know the message is sinking in.

At these assemblies, a video is shown, typically of students at a party and then someone gets into a car to drive another home. Always, as in real life, the drunk driver is not hurt, just very confused, and his passenger and friend is killed. These videos, projected onto a large screen for the assembly, show the partying, the decision to drive drunk, a crashed car, the Jaws of Life to extract the body from the car, the arrest of the drunk driver, the doctors working on the seriously hurt student, the death, and then the parent notification. These programs are very powerful. After all of this, the "dead" students read their letters as if they were dead and parents read their letters about their "dead" children to the school. After the assemblies, the "dead" students can once again be with their parents and friends in a very emotional reunion.

Not long after I got out of the hospital–about six months after the accident–my parents took me to the engineering firm where I used to work as the Marketing Communications Specialist so I could have lunch with my old boss and several others. When I left that day, I tried to give my key back, and they wouldn't let me. What a generous gesture–at that time, the best I could do was to work on remembering the names of my brother's mechanical engineering master's courses ("Control Feedback Design") and push myself to use both hands typing my email. I was right-handed before the accident, but now my left hand is more functional.

So I struggle with what my new career will be. I decided that I need to do something that matters, and so I will continue giving my presentation to students of all ages and to the cadets at the California Highway Patrol (CHP) Academy. Occasionally the hard-to-impress high school audiences will gasp when they see the photographs of my smashed bike, a signal that I may have had an impact. At another high school, one student complained loudly that "he only got eight years!?"

The children from my old doctor's child's elementary school, Cottage Hill in Alta Sierra, asked a lot of questions. Then something I loved happened–about 30 first-through-third grade students simply lined up and each gave me a hug, saying "thank you" as they embraced me. I was dumbfounded—feeling like they really heard me, despite their young ages.

Just as wonderful, sometimes the new CHP cadets

who've heard me speak will email me after they make their first driving-under-the-influence arrest. They've written that they made the arrest in my name. That makes me feel like my talks have had an impact and may have spared some unknown lives the loss and devastation caused by a drunk driver.

But I need to do more. I've been volunteering in local elementary schools, helping children learning English as a second language. I volunteer for the physical therapy students at Sacramento State each semester so I am able to teach them about working with real patients with physical limitations, rather than simply reading about it. I also take physical education classes four times a week at American River and Sac City colleges to keep up my strength.

I don't know what the next step is. I have disability insurance and social security to cover my basic expenses, but additional income would be good. Most important, I've got to feel productive. I'm not sure what to expect because I'm totally different than I was before. What I do know is that I need to be doing something with people directly, not the marketing communications like I was doing before my injury. Since my head injury, I make decisions more slowly, but once made, I am pretty fiercely focused. Once I decided I was moving out of my parents' home, I was very set on reaching my goal. Now I just need to figure out a new path to a career. The occupations I'm interested in now deal more with people, rather that the written word. But because of my head injury, I am not about to go back to school to get another master's degree; my memory is not made for school anymore.

▪   ▪   ▪

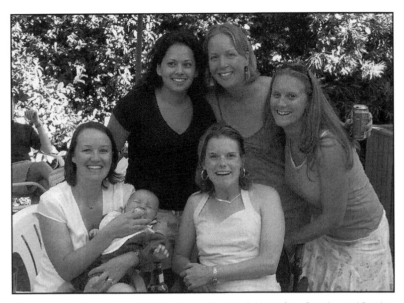

Jill surrounded by friends Heidi (with son Thomas), Veronica, Sarah, and Becky.

CHAPTER FIFTEEN

LOVE

"Now and then it is good to pause in our pursuit of happiness and just be happy."
Guillaume Apollinaire

One of the only temporary blessings of the early months after the injury was that I couldn't remember Alan. My body and my brain and my heart were so overwhelmed that it may have been a good thing I didn't have to cope with losing him, too. Not knowing what I remembered or understood, my parents decided not to mention him at all until I did. When I started to go through emails and websites four months after the accident I grasped somewhat fleetingly that there had been an even larger loss. One of the emails I saw mentioned a service that was being held to pray for my recovery and to remember Alan.

A year after the accident, I started a new journal, and my first entry was about missing Alan. My memories of him had finally returned in force. Sometimes I played the game with his spirit: if I had the choice of meeting you and having this happen to me or never meeting you and still being mobile, I would choose you. I wrote him letters full of love and full of sadness and full of anger about my new life sentence. I talked with him.

Letters that I wrote to him and those I wrote from him helped, even though they were hard. Talking helped.

Some days were—and are—worse than others. When I close my eyes, I can still see him opening the door just a tiny crack after my knock. Through the crack, I can only see one of his luminous eyes, and he peeks out and whispers "hi." He wrote me and told me he thought we were meant for each other. I wonder if there will ever be a man who could possibly have his heart, his energy, his stoicism, his athleticism, and his love of life. Anyone even close would have to be amazing, and that makes me scared for anyone in my future. Sometimes I despair, not only missing Alan, but missing the promise of our life together. In our conversations, earth-to-heaven, he sometimes tells me he's trying to find someone like him who I can love again, but typically, he tells me that it's up to me to find him. "Don't be complacent," he says. "You've overcome so much, but you can do more."

When I swim at the pool, I imagine what he would be saying to me when I get scared to put my face under without plugging my nose. Alan would probably be going nuts watching my mistakes knowing he could, with a word, make me better than I am. "Don't be afraid," he would say from his perch next to heaven's pool, "go ahead and put your face in the water." He would be looking on the bright side, telling me how every lane up there is the fast lane. I promise him I will work to make him happy and proud. A coach and a lover, he tells me, "Meet your goals because you want to be happy, not because you want me to be happy. And I'm already so proud of you." In the pool is where we first connected, and he loved the water so much, so it makes sense that in the water is when I think of him especially often.

More than two years after the accident, I met Alan's newborn nephew, Gabe. I was worried he was going to look like Alan, but it turned out that it was far more difficult to look into his sister's eyes so exactly like his. Even her facial expressions brought him back. I thought at the time that I couldn't understand how his parents managed being reminded all the time of his beautiful face. I missed him more than ever. I was sad that Gabe would never know his uncle and would never have his uncle's advice on swimming and playing basketball and how to respect other people and how to live. I hoped Alan was looking out for his little nephew, like he does me; we have the best guardian angel.

More than three years after the accident, my brother and I went to a Mountain View Masters swim meet and then had lunch at Le Bou where Alan and I used to eat breakfast sometimes after swimming. After lunch, we drove by Alan's old condominium. I originally thought I wanted to get out of the car and peek inside, but the windows were covered with white wooden blinds that weren't Alan's. Alan, finally, wasn't there. I cried as we drove out of the parking lot, following the path we used to run together. The crying helped.

One of my friends at school said he didn't stop missing his girlfriend until he found someone new. For me, I think this is a vital piece of information. I miss Alan every day. Sometimes, I find myself crying when I'm alone, seemingly for no reason, but it's always about losing him. In the summer of 2008, I finally went to see where his ashes are in Berkeley. My parents came with me to the cemetery. I wasn't sure I wanted to go, but I'm glad I did. I needed to see. I left him a perfect sunflower. Not long after, I had a dream. Alan spoke to me, the first time since he died. When I woke up, though, and realized he was gone, I cried. He wanted me to know, though, that he liked the man I was dating at the time.

I met him at a sports class at American River College in Sacramento. We got to know each other as we wheeled around the gym together, doing laps, and he taught me better techniques for wheeling my chair faster. Because he has been paralyzed since he was 17 (he's my age), he was an expert on a lot of things I needed to know. The thing I like about him is that he does not use his disability as a barrier for anything. Two people in wheelchairs have some unique challenges. The first night he asked me out, he rolled me to my car after our class and then asked if he could see me sometime. Ignoring the romantic aspects, I immediately leapt to the practical and asked him how that would work. How, for instance, would we get both our chairs into one car? We didn't for the first date, but we figured it out later.

I think I am, finally, ready to open my heart. Sometimes I think: Who would want to date someone in a wheelchair with a brain injury? My confidence was definitely hurt along with my ability to feel sexy. Once when I was driving with Christy in Grass Valley, we noticed a guy in the car glancing over at us. "He's checking you out!" she said. I snapped back that he didn't know I was in a chair. She never let me forget how foolish that comment was.

Sometimes people say that only I could deal with a life change like this, and they ask, "How do you do it?" Not many people could do what I've done, they say to me. But lots of people do and lots of people can. We've got no other choice than to make the best of what has happened. And I want to make Alan's friends and family proud he was with a fighter. So I fight.

. . .

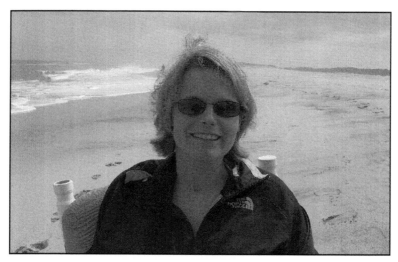

Jill at Assateague National Seashore, Maryland, in 2008.

CHAPTER SIXTEEN

BECOMING MYSELF

"In my philosophy/belief system, nothing happens 'by accident.' Everything happens on purpose, for a reason—even though that reason may be obscured, sometimes for years. Events that seem horrible at the onset turn out to be necessary lessons that are blessings in disguise. One not only learns to accept them, but eventually to embrace and be grateful for them because the growth and wisdom they provoke wouldn't or couldn't have occurred otherwise."

Sally Mason

In some ways I am like a teenager trying to find herself again. Who am I? How changed am I? What does the future hold?

I went to my ten-year high school reunion in 2005, and it was a trip. I went with several of my friends from high school and, luckily, I was able to warn everyone on the electronic invitation that I would be rolling up. However, for people who did not know about my injury, they asked me about Alan. Man. I should have explained that as well but did not want to put something so serious on an electronic invitation. Several of my friends met at my parents' house before so we could go together. At the reunion, we pretty much stayed at our table, and a lot of folks came up to talk; it was fun to see everyone.

Since moving to Sacramento and living independently, I've joined a few spinal cord injury groups. The groups are mostly too conservative for me in the sense that the participants seem surprised by the "normal" things I do. You sleep in a normal bed? You drive a sedan and not a van? I was surprised to find myself feeling a kind of prejudice against paralyzed people who manage to take what happened to them and use it to make excuses for their behaviors or lack of action. Then I realized my prejudices haven't changed at all–I've never liked to be around whining.

There's no getting around some pretty big changes, though. I don't have the stamina I used to. It takes me forever to get ready. I'm always cold. My education doesn't seem to matter sometimes. I get frustrated and sad, something I never struggled with before. I feel like snapping at people who say, with all good intentions, "It's nice to see you out." "What should I do?" I think. "Stay home all day because I am in a chair? Or "Is it that bad to let people see me out in my chair?' "They let you out," I'd like to say, "why can't I be out, too?" I, of course, say none of the above. They actually have a very small point because it is harder for me to get out than it was before. The littlest things can make me tired. The other day I napped for two-and-a-half hours. I hate it that getting dressed, showering, getting into a car, and even going to bed tire me out. People will ask me what I did that day, and, often, the answer is "I don't know!" when I was busy all day! This is a combination of the head injury and the fact that it takes me so much longer to do the simplest things.

I have learned to limit my commitments. Compromising is something I end up doing all of the time. Pre-accident, I would drive all over the Bay Area, from Mountain View to Grass Valley, at the drop of a hat. I can't do that anymore. I can't do nearly as much in a day as I could before. What's actually frightening is that I am not minding as much, maybe because the realization has come with an appreciation for the smaller things in life I used to take for granted. It also may be maturity. Maybe I would have been like this anyway. In any case, I try to be more succinct, aware as I am of the preciousness of time.

Buying my car–and not a van–provoked an identify crisis of sorts. Would I be a van person? I found myself increasingly irritated with people who assumed I couldn't manage anything else. I sought out other people in chairs who had chosen differently and offered good advice about what kind of sedans work best.

My sports groups that I joined at Sacramento's American River College are full of people who are in wheelchairs and not whining. What has been important is to keep taking courses, keep looking for groups. One group that's wrong for me will be right for someone else. You just have to keep going back at it.

Of course, I am, admittedly, splendidly lucky to have my family. It goes without saying that I could not have functioned–would not be functioning–without my parents and my brother, but there are so many others. My grammy, my aunts, my uncles, and my cousins, all of whom continue to help me. Jess, a close cousin in age, and her husband Josh live only about 10 minutes away now; they even have a key to my house so they can come in and pick me up off the floor if necessary.

Even as I struggle with my own identity, I am at least sure I don't want to be one of those people who use their disability as an identity. Someone said once that she had done more in her chair than out. I am the opposite of that: at this point I feel as if I have done more out of my chair than in and I know what it is like to run, to feel the sand on my toes, to sweat. It's very mixed up sometimes, though.

OLYMPIC TORCHBEARING

In April of 2008, nearly four years to the day of the accident, I carried the Olympic torch through the streets of San Francisco. This is something I wouldn't have done before the accident. A visitor to my website, Jen Mayor, asked me to submit an essay entry to be considered. I did and then forgot about it until I was notified of my selection. In spite of the protesters and the last-minute changes to the route that kept my family and friends from seeing me in person (they saw me on television) with the official torch, I was completely thrilled to be involved. Some of the local media interviewed me. Dan was with me in the van following; we had a grand time.

To be considered for the honor, I sent the following essay to the Olympic committee:

"I received a request to my website (www.jillmason. com) to submit an entry to carry the Olympic Torch in San Francisco. I was flattered and surprised. On Easter Sunday, April 11, 2004, at 11:30 a.m., my boyfriend Alan and I were hit on a training bike ride by a driver who was four times the legal limit drunk. Alan was killed instantly; and I am now a wheelchair user with a head injury. Alan and I were so happy—swimming, riding, and running together and competing in triathlons. To help prevent this from happening to others, I give PowerPoint presentations to schools and am involved in the "Every 15 Minutes" program at high schools. (Every 15 minutes is the average time in which someone is killed by a drunk driver.) So what sustains me when so much of what I loved is now gone? I have a wonderful family. I love teaching students about the dangers of drinking and driving. I'm writing a book to help others who have had or know someone who's had a life-changing event. I should be considered to carry the torch in San Francisco to show that nobody should let one devastating experience change his attitude towards life."

The whole experience was insane. My brother Dan was my buddy the whole time. We had the torchbearers' reception the night before at the Chinese Art Museum in San Francisco. We met many of the other torchbearers and mingled with former Olympians, the head of Olympic Security (who had just returned from and was traveling back to Beijing), and former San Francisco mayor Willie Brown. Dan and I really felt like we did not belong there. He quickly put on a nice jacket because I erroneously said he'd be fine without one. The current San Francisco mayor Gavin Newsom gave a speech to the attendees in one of the fancier rooms, and then we headed back to our hotel. Several of my mom's students from Union Hill made congratulatory posters for me that my parents hung all over our hotel room. It was very sweet and really sort of brought everything into reality.

The next morning, we went to breakfast then down to the torchbearers' orientation in one of the big conference rooms at the hotel. Once again, we mingled with former Olympians, stars, politicians, and heads of security. Gavin Newsom stood on top of a table to give his last words of wisdom prior to us departing for the two buses and my van.

It was pretty funny because the way they affixed my torch holder to my wheelchair was with this metal bar and duck tape. (They used Dan's engineering expertise, of course.) So, Dan, our driver, and my escort were led to my van and then we sat. We sat for about two hours twiddling our thumbs, waiting for the motorcade to make a move. Then, we saw Gavin Newsom in a huddle with all the head security guys behind my van. It finally looked like something was happening. After two-plus hours of hanging out, the motorcycle cops started screaming down the sidewalks on each side of the road.

Meanwhile, my family and some of my friends were waiting along the Embarcadero where I was supposed to carry the torch. They watched as protesters stormed a fake bus. The officials sent out a sort of trial balloon bus to see what would happen, and it's a good thing they did.

We started driving! Then, while along Van Ness Avenue, the bus in front of us started letting torchbearers out! We still had no idea what we were doing. Only when one of the chief guys came to my van when we were along the Marina and said it was time to go, did I know where I was carrying the torch. (And, thank goodness it was flat!) As I was unloading off the van, a dude with a black pillow case over his face stood in front of a van about 50 yards away from me. Immediately, I was surrounded by probably 10 cops. It was quite scary. The person was not violent, but trying to stop the progression. Once he was taken away, I met up with my two torchbearing buddies and we transferred the flame from the other torchbearers to our torch. I pushed for about 50 feet and then we decided it was easier for someone else to push me. It all happened so fast.

Then, the torch was gone, and so was the bus. Dan found me and I had a policeman by me, and that was it. So, here we were, like sitting ducks in the middle of the road. Finally, my van found me and we drove back to the hotel where I was to get my torch. (I was starving because it was about 3 p.m., and I had not had a chance to have lunch, so one of my many aunts who were there bought me a mini pizza from the hotel restaurant.)

When the bus arrived back from the send off ceremony at the San Francisco airport, everyone went over to a little room in the hotel where we each got a real torch that had been lit by the Olympic flame! (I did not go to the send off ceremonies because even my drivers were clueless about where they had moved the send-off ceremony.) Overall, it was an amazing experience.

FINAL THOUGHTS

One old friend said to me: "You aren't defined by your chair, you just use one to get around." I liked that. It was a refreshing way to look at my predicament. I like to follow Allen Rucker's advice: don't let your paralysis dominate conversations. Curiously, though, people tend to discuss their pains with me, thinking I will understand because I'm paralyzed. Hmm. Fact is I don't have any pain, which is unbelievable when you think about the surgery I went through.

I've also turned into one of those people who goes crazy seeing a handicapped placard misused or a car idling in a handicapped spot. They don't realize that we can't park there–and we have to have a spot with enough room to get our chairs out and re-assembled, not to speak about not having to roll miles to the entrance.

I'm not in traumatic brain injury groups because the range of recovery is so varied. I haven't yet found a group of people with similar goals: keep going, make something out of your disrupted life, make plans for the future.

At the same time I've been coping with major life changes caused by the accident, I've begun to notice that my friends and I are going through some other more routine cosmic shifts. My friends from college have developed their own lives, and our relationships have changed, just as they would have whether or not I were in a chair. We've all made friends in our new lives constrained by geography and other choices. I made a lot of those growing-up decisions all over again and in radically changed circumstances.

On days I feel sorry for myself and am depressed, I can't ponder the future at all. I'm focused on putting on my shoes and getting my chair and person in the car, and working or relationships are simply outside my scope. Then I get mad at the one man, Harvey, who caused all the bad things. But I move on, because at my core I can't waste too much time being angry. My hope is that I can help another family face what we've faced.

Now that I am done with this book, it is sort of a catch-22. I am thrilled to be finished after all of the years of recalling funny, painful, and memorable stories. Yet my own story, dealing with the aftermath of one man's actions, is never going to end. However, I am not able to end on a sad note because that is not who I am at my core. In writing this, I have realized that there is no way I would be able to handle everything that has happened if it weren't for the wonderful upbringing I was lucky enough to have had.

My dad's cousin's words dog me. She wondered if I had found any unexpected growth and wisdom in "the years since your life was shattered and derailed so horribly, and so unfairly" while "on a path you never thought to tread." Or wanted to tread. Yes, I have to say, though it's still early days. "You certainly are doing wondrous things." I'd like to do wondrous things, and I'd like to help someone else, even if I can't know that I am, and even if I'm not sure I can. This is not a path I chose. But I have to make the best of it.

And I hope to find myself again.

. . .

ADDENDA

A. Addendum: How to Find Helpful and Hopeful Information

Websites

Jill Mason
www.JillMason.com

My hope is that my own website–begun by my brother and my friend Danh a few days after the accident–will give some hope to families because it shows my progress, especially in the photo gallery.

Spinal Cord Injury
National Spinal Cord Injury Association (NSCIA)
www.spinalcord.org/

I didn't see a lot of helpful information for me on this site, but it seems to be the leading organization and lobby for people with SCI. It's been around for sixty years.

Traumatic Brain Injury
Traumatic Brain Injury Survival Guide
http://www.tbiguide.com

U.S. Government Center for Disease Control (CDC) National Center for Injury Prevention and Control: What is Traumatic

Brain Injury?

http://www.cdc.gov/ncipc/tbi/TBI.htm

This government page provides a wealth of free information and links to research, data, and tips. CDC even provides occasional podcasts.

National Institute of Neurological Disorders and Stroke (NINDS)

http://www.ninds.nih.gov/disorders/tbi/tbi.htm

National Institute of Neurological Disorders and Stroke (NINDS), part of the National Institutes of Health, links to a number of other helpful organizations. "NINDS conducts and supports research on brain and nervous system disorders. Created by the U.S. Congress in 1950."

Brain Injury Association of America (BIAA)

http://www.biausa.org

"Founded in 1980, the Brain Injury Association of America (BIAA) is the leading national organization serving and representing individuals, families and professionals who are touched by a life-altering, often devastating, traumatic brain injury (TBI). Together with its network of more than 40 chartered state affiliates, as well as hundreds of local chapters and support groups across the country, the BIAA provides information, education and support to assist the 5.3 million Americans currently living with traumatic brain injury and their families."

Books
Spinal Cord Injury
Medical/Professional Guidance

Palmer, Sara, Kriegsman, Kay Harris, and Palmer, Jeffrey B., **Spinal Cord Injury: A Guide for Living (A Johns Hopkins Press Health Book),** The Johns Hopkins University Press; second edition, 2008

Written by rehabilitation professionals, this book helps chart treatments and choices during recovery. Well-organized with chapters and sections that can be read separately.

First-person Accounts

Rucker, Allen, **The Best Seat in the House: How I Woke Up One Tuesday and Was Paralyzed for Life**, HarperCollins, 2007

Suddenly paralyzed from the waste down by transverse myelitis, television writer Allen Rucker provides a great, non-whining glimpse into the ten years he's spent adapting to life in a wheelchair.

Willette, Kate, **Some Things are Unbreakable**, Lulu. com, 2007

The wife of an skiing accident victim, Kate Willette writes about their first year post-accident tackling hope and despair and and abundance of medical technology.

Traumatic Brain Injury
Medical/Professional Guidance

Senelick, Richard C. and Dougherty, Karla, **Living with Brain Injury: A Guide for Families**, CENGAGE Delmar Learning,

2nd edition, 2001

First-person Accounts

Swanson, Kara L., **I'll Carry the Fork! Recovering Life After Brain Injury**, Rising Star Press, 1999

Kara Swanson tells her difficult story of life following a serious car accident with great humor. An easy read that explains a lot to family members.

Osborn, Claudia L., **Over My Head: A Doctor's Own Story of Head Injury from the Inside Looking Out**, Andrews McMeel Publishing, 2nd edition 2000

Physician Claudia Osborn writes simply about the devastating effects of TBI from the patient's point of view—her own—as she works to recover from a bike accident. An excellent book for families struggling to understand the cognitive and personality changes that may endure.

Meili, Trisha, **I Am the Central Park Jogger: A Story of Hope and Possibility**, Scribner 2004

Trisha Meili was brutally beaten, raped, sodomized and left for dead in Central Park in 1989. She tells how she learned again to talk, feed herself, think, and walk. My girlfriends shared this book just after my accident.

Taylor, Jill Bolte, **My Stroke of Insight: A Brain Scientist's Personal Journey**, Viking, 2008

While Jill Taylor's stroke was not the result of an injury, she describes from the inside (and as a scientist) how it feels to have a brain that functions differently from the one you had before.

Hope

Tresniowski, Alex, **When Life Gives You Lemons: Remarkable Stories of People Overcoming Adversity**, McGraw-Hill Companies, 1st edition 2000.

Inspirational stories of people whose names you've heard and those you haven't who overcame serious challenges and regained lives.

Fumia, Molly, **Safe Passage: Words to Help the Grieving,** Conari Press; New Ed edition, 2003

Exactly what the title conveys: Molly Fumia's words are comforting in the face of terrible losses.

Articles about Jill Mason

CYCLIST KILLED, 1 HURT ON HWY. 12; Published on April 12, 2004; © 2004- The Press Democrat; BYLINE: KATY HILLENMEYER; PAGE: B1

SONOMA COUNTY: **Widespread ripples extend from fatal crash; Damage to families of slain bicyclist, badly injured friend**; San Francisco Chronicle; by Ryan Kim, Pamela J. Podger and Peter Fimrite, Chronicle Staff Writers; Monday, April 19, 2004; on www.sfisonline.com

SJSU alumna, paralyzed in April accident, released from hospital; 'She had a joyful outlook on life that was infectious.' by Ling-Mei Wong, Spartan Daily (San Jose State University, CA); Issue date: 9/20/04 on //www.thespartandaily.com/

SANTA ROSA: **Drunken driver gets prison; He hit cyclists – man killed, woman injured**; San Francisco Chronicle; by Pamela J. Podger, Chronicle Staff Writer; Tuesday, September 28, 2004; on www.sfgate.com

SANTA ROSA MAN GETS NEARLY 9 YEARS IN KILLING OF BICYCLIST ON HWY. 12; Published on September 28, 2004 © 2004- The Press Democrat; BYLINE: STEVE HART; PAGE: A1

Racing toward recovery; Jill Mason works to overcome injuries from drunken driver; Union (Grass Valley, CA); By David Mirhadi; Wednesday, November 23, 2005; on www.theunion.com

Olympic torchbearers of San Francisco, Sustainable Journeys Essay Contest; San Francisco Chronicle website; April 4, 2008; on www.sfgate.com

Torchbearer's Essay, Jill Mason, Sacramento; San Francisco Chronicle website; April 4, 2008; on www.sfgate.com

Carry the Torch; Santa Clara University Alumni Magazine; Summer 2008; by Steven Boyd Saum; on www.scu.edu/scm

Broken by David Darlington

Excerpted from Bicycling Magazine, January 2008.

Reprinted with permission of the publisher and the author.

ON EASTER SUNDAY OF 2004, Alan Liu and Jill Mason embarked on a bike ride from Santa Rosa. They'd been dating for about six months since meeting on the master's swim team in Mountain View, south of San Francisco. Liu, 31, was the team's head coach; a graduate of MIT and Stanford, he was employed by Applied Materials, a semiconductor-equipment manufacturer in Silicon Valley, where he'd recently been made a manager. (He also held four engineering patents.) In addition, Liu was a successful coach: A competitive swimmer since age five, he was known for encouraging people to perform beyond their own expectations. Since taking over the 300- member Mountain View master's program in 1997, he'd expanded it to include water polo and triathlons.

Like Liu, Mason, 26, was a triathlete. Growing up in the -Sierra Nevada foothills, she'd been a member of the track, cross-country, lacrosse and soccer teams at Nevada Union High School, where she was nicknamed Forrest Gump because of her surprising speed. Shorter than most of her opponents, Mason was a fierce competitor in the 100-meter hurdles despite taking four steps between each set of barriers instead of the usual three (and thus leading with a different leg on every other hurdle). She had gone on to run marathons at Santa Clara University, which she'd attended at the same time as Ross Dillon-in fact, she'd contributed to his rehabilitation fund the previous year. With a new master's degree in mass communications from San Jose State, Mason was working as a marketing director for an environmental and geotechnical engineering company in Mountain View, where she met Alan Liu after joining the swim team. The confident, upbeat Mason was a match for the energetic Liu, and soon the two of them were running, riding and swimming together regularly.

They planned their Easter ride to prepare for an upcoming half- Ironman triathlon, riding 30 miles in Sonoma Valley that April 11, passing not far from the Dillons' house on Trinity Road. At 11:19 a.m., the route brought them back into eastern Santa Rosa on California Highway 12, a high-speed artery that becomes increasingly congested as it approaches the city. Local riders avoid it, but Liu and Mason were out-of-town visitors, seeking the most direct route back into town to meet Liu's mother for brunch.

As the couple pedaled west on the highway, Harvey Hereford got into his Nissan Sentra at the seniors-only Oakmont subdivision, adjacent to Highway 12. Hereford wasn't expecting any Easter visitors; on the contrary, he later said that he felt deserted by his family. A 69-year-old personal-injury attorney, he was described by neighbors as a friendly and funny guy, but his ex-wife had recently called police when she couldn't reach him, thinking he might be suicidal. Over the past 15 years, 10 federal tax liens and one state Employment Development lien had been issued against

Hereford's office and former residence in San Francisco.

At 11:20, a pair of Oakmont residents, Kate Brolan and Sydney Brown, were sitting in their car on Pythian Road, waiting at a red light at the intersection with Highway 12. When the light turned green, a Nissan Sentra in front of them pulled out and turned toward Santa Rosa; within seconds, according to Brown, it was flying "like a shot out of hell," weaving all over the road as it bore down on a pair of cyclists on the shoulder. Liu was riding behind Mason, and the car hit him first, killing him instantly as it severed his brain stem. An instant later it slammed into Mason, cleaving her spinal cord, lacerating her liver, breaking her arm and traumatizing her brain. When Brolan and Brown reached her, she was sobbing and shivering on the ground.

Not unlike Cathie Hamer's Mitsubishi, the Nissan came to a stop a hundred yards up the road, where its driver was detained by a couple of passing off-duty cops. -Hereford, whose driver's license was found to have expired, told the officers that he suspected something was wrong when he noticed that his windshield was broken. He didn't remember running into anybody; nor did he remember getting into his car or driving away from his house. His blood-alcohol percentage was 0.29, more than three times the legal limit.

As with Ross Dillon, doctors at Santa Rosa Memorial Hospital expected Mason to either die or remain in a vegetative state. A day after the crash, her mother and father - Joanne, a school counselor, and Larry, an adaptive phys ed teacher for disabled students-were given the same pessimistic advice the Dillons had received. That night, more than three dozen Sonoma County Bicycle Coalition members gathered in front of the county courthouse and rode in silence to the hospital, where they held a candlelight vigil for Mason. Among them were Betsy and Rusty Dillon, who urged Mason's parents not to give up-they said they'd received similar predictions about Ross, and that two years later he was still improving.

Sure enough, the next day Jill Mason's doctors reported that her prognosis wasn't as bad as they'd feared. But the story was over for Alan Liu, whose stepsister had been killed by a drunk driver on New Year's Day the previous year.

. . .

B. ADDENDUM: RECOVERY TIMELINE

April 11, 2004: Harvey Hereford hits Jill Mason and Alan Liu as they are biking in Santa Rosa, California; Alan is killed, and she is critically injured.

Santa Rosa Memorial Hospital

April 12, 2004: Some major swelling down, critical portions of brain thought to be damaged were probably not; response to nerve stimulation test good

April 14, 2004: Opened both eyes; blood pressure not as high; bruising of lungs and infection diagnosed; turns out to be fluid caught behind a lung

April 18, 2004: Completely off the ventilator

April 20, 2004: Infection, probably in her lungs

April 21, 2004: Surgery begins at 0730; lasts 12 hours; surgeons set major dislocation in her back

April 22, 2004: Only response to verbal or physical contact was slight elevation of hr and blood pressure; no eye opening

April 23, 2004: Woke up briefly, but level of consciousness seems much less advanced than pre-surgery.

April 24, 2004: Fever broke, but little responsiveness

April 25, 2004: Santa Clara and Grass Valley events

April 25, 2004: Alan's funeral service

April 25, 2004: Right side of body tense possibly because of brain swelling in her temporal lobe; stuck out her tongue; family told recovery process for this type of head injury extremely long and uncertain

April 26, 2004: Nose tube and some others gone; completely off morphine; alertness higher, but response to verbal commands still not as good pre-surgery; plans made to move to Santa Clara rehab in a week or two

April 28, 2004: Doctor says she responded to a verbal command for the first time since surgery; she yawns; brief dip in O2 levels, but probably just some fluid

April 29, 2004: Extended tense/spastic right arm on her own and opened her hand for her mother; shows facial expressions; breathing pattern deeper and more relaxed

April 30, 2004: Moved fingers on command for doctors

May 2, 2004: Wildflower Triathlon; Saturday race dedicated to Alan, a race Sunday dedicated to Jill's recovery

May 2, 2004: Three states documented: 20-40% sleeping, 40-50% extremely uncomfortable; 20-30% aware and seems to enjoy her family, making eye contact, following motion, even smiling

Santa Clara Valley Medical Center

May 13, 2004: Transferred by ambulance to Santa Clara Valley Medical Center

May 16, 2004: Spinal fluid culture cloudy; no responsiveness

May 20, 2004: Shunt removed and replaced with ventriculostomy

May 20, 2004: Small pockets of fluid in liver found; were infected, later drained

May 27, 2004: EEG: vacant stare record showing generalized slowing but increased activity with stimulation

May 28, 2004: Family care conference predicted "small chance of independence"; continues agitated and unresponsive

June 1, 2004: Clamped shunt to see if handling pressure

June 9, 2004: Another shunt operation; cut all my hair off

June 13, 2004: Read simple commands

June 14, 2004: Removed neck collar

June 15, 2004: Removed Foley catheter and began intermittent catheterization

June 17, 2004: Ate ice chips

June 21, 2004: Said "Hi, Mom," in a whispery, squeaky voice

June 25, 2004: Using 4-5 word sentences like "I want to go home," "Where is the car?"

June 26, 2004: Drank cranberry juice by holding cup; brought to mouth with minimal assistance

June 27, 2004: Wrote first and last name and her brother's name, underlining his

July 3, 2004: Initiating requests, asking about dinner

July 6-10, 2004: Eating pureed foods

July 12, 2004: Beginning to eat real food with spoon and fork

July 12, 2004: Pushing wheelchair using weak left arm five feet for about 45 seconds

July 23, 2004: First outing in van to a restaurant with other patients, and first time asking about who Alan's mom was

July 23, 2004: Can balance with both hands in seated position

July 27, 2004: Emailed Daniel, Mom and Dad using left index finger; remembered email addresses

August 20, 2004: To sushi for lunch and then to Los Gatos downtown for picnic in the park in the evening

August 28, 2004: Pass to visit Sarah for lunch in Santa Cruz

September 4, 2004: Jill tells Dan what to write on website; thanks everyone

September 4, 2004: Cleared for a normal diet

September, 2004: Once cleared for normal diet, speech therapist Theresa takes Jill to the kitchen to select food

September 5, 2004: Pass to go to Grammy's for the day in Marin County

Starting Over: Going Home to Grass Valley

September 14, 2004: Leaves Santa Clara Valley Medical Center in San Jose to move to Grass Valley

September 17 or 18, 2004: Karaoke and Auction night at a bar in downtown Grass Valley

September 27: Sentencing hearing for Harvey Hereford in Santa Rosa

October, November, December, 2004: Tuesday-Wednesday-Thursday therapy schedule

October 4, 2004: Tackling the Independence Trail with aunt and uncle Paula and Bill and Dan, a wheelchair accessible trail by the south fork of the Yuba Riva; pushed myself for half hour

October 11, 2004: First new wheelchair; doesn't fit, too heavy

October 14, 2004: Original neurosurgeon from Santa Rosa indicates independence just might be possible

October 20, 2004: Return to Lowney to visit with friends and go to Monterey

November 12, 2004: New titanium wheelchair arrives; working on bed transfers

December 13, 2004: New attendant, Christy, arrives, replacing disastrous daily attendants

January 2005: Took brain test at UC Davis Medical Center that predicted driving and independence were not likely

December 2005: Organized holiday party slide show with Erin for former engineering firm

Independence: Moving to Sacramento

August 26, 2006: Moved into apartment in Sacramento with roommate

September 1 2007: Article in Sacramento Bee

October 7, 2006: Hospital stay of three days for infected heel begins

October 2006: First long plane trip to Vermont and New York

April 9, 2008: Carried Olympic torch through the streets of
San Francisco; selected through an essay contest

July 2008: Bought a house in South Sacramento;
realtor's husband was the contractor who did most
modifications.

September 2008: Hospitalized for 4 days at UC Davis for
pressure sore

Present: Continues to give speeches to high schools on impact
of drunk driving and takes P.E. classes at Sacramento
City College

■ ■ ■

C. ADDENDUM: JILL'S FAVORITE QUOTES

"A pessimist sees the difficulty in every opportunity; an optimist sees the opportunity in every difficulty." Sir Winston Churchill

"Not everything that can be counted counts, and not everything that counts can be counted." Albert Einstein

"If you are out to describe the truth, leave elegance to the tailor." Albert Einstein

"The best and safest thing is to keep a balance in your life, acknowledge the great powers around us and in us. If you can do that, and live that way, you are really a wise man." Euripides

"Slight not what's near, while aiming at what's far." Euripides, 'Rhesus'

"Dost thou love life? Then do not squander time; for that's the stuff life is made of." Benjamin Franklin

"The toughest opponent of all is Old Man Par. He's a patient soul who never shoots a birdie and never incurs a bogey. And if you would travel the long road with him, you must be patient, too." Bobby Tyre Jones

"Whenever you are asked if you can do a job, tell 'em, 'Certainly, I can!' Then get busy and find out how to do it." Theodore Roosevelt

"Stop a moment, cease your work, look around you." Leo Tolstoy

"When you cannot get a compliment any other way, pay yourself one." Mark Twain

"It often shows a find command of language to say nothing." Anonymous

"Pains of love be sweeter far more than all other pleasures are." John Dryden

"A content person enjoys scenery on a detour." Anonymous

"The will to win means nothing without the will to prepare." Juma Ikangaa

"Love is the only game that is not called on account of darkness." Thomas Carlyle

"Appreciation is like salt—a little goes a long way to bring out the best in us." Anonymous

"Never let yesterday use up too much of today." Will Rogers

"Expose yourself to your greatest fear, after that, fear has no power, and the fear of freedom shrinks and vanishes." Jim Morrison

"Money will buy a fine dog, but only love will make it wag its tail." Richard Friedman

"An eye for an eye leaves the whole world blind." Mahatma Gandhi

"The real voyage of discovery consists not in seeking new landscapes, but in having new eyes." Marcel Proust

"Remember the tea kettle-it is always up to its neck in hot water, yet it still sings." Anonymous

"But to see her was to love her, love but her, and love her forever." Robert Burns

"You have to do your own growing, no matter how tall your grandfather was." Abraham Lincoln

"Now and then it is good to pause in our pursuit of happiness and just be happy." Guillaume Apollinaire

"A friend is the first person who comes in when the world has gone out." Anonymous

"Love is the only thing that can be divided without being diminished." Anonymous

"Enjoy the little things, for one day you may discover they were the big things." Robert Brault

"A true test of character is not how much we know how to do, but how we behave when we don't know what to do." John W. Holt, Jr.

"All the flowers of all the tomorrows are in the seeds of today." Anonymous

"The journey of a thousand miles begins with a single step." Confucius

"Muddy water, let stand, becomes clear." Lao Tzu

"You'll learn more about the road by traveling it than consulting all the maps in the world." Unknown

"Celebrate, we will, because life is short but sweet for
certain." Dave Matthews

"Where there is great love there, are always miracles."
Willa Cather